ISSUES IN BI

Health and the Good Society

The goals of healthcare and health policy, and the health-related dilemmas facing policy makers, professionals, and citizens are extensively analysed and debated in a range of disciplines including public health, sociology, and applied philosophy. *Health and the Good Society* is the first full-length work that addresses these debates in a way that cuts across these disciplinary boundaries.

Alan Cribb's core argument is that clinical ethics needs to be understood in the context of public health ethics. This entails healthcare ethics embracing 'the social dimension' of health in two overlapping senses: first, the various respects in which health experiences and outcomes are socially determined; and second, the ways in which health-related goods are better understood as social rather then purely individual goods. This broader approach to the ethics of healthcare includes a concern with the social construction of both healthcare goods and the roles, ideals, and obligations of agents; that is to say it focuses upon the 'value field' of health-related action and not only upon the ethics of action within this value field. This ground-breaking book thus seeks to 'open up' the agenda of healthcare ethics both methodologically and substantively: it argues that population-oriented perspectives are central to all healthcare ethics, and that everybody has some share of responsibility for securing health-related goods including the good of greater health equality. One of its major conclusions is that the rather limited tradition of health education policy and practice needs to be completely rethought.

Alan Cribb is Professor of Bioethics and Education at the Centre for Public Policy Research, King's College London.

ISSUES IN BIOMEDICAL ETHICS

General Editors
John Harris and Søren Holm

Consulting Editors
Raanan Gillon and Bonnie Steinbock

The late twentieth century witnessed dramatic technological developments in biomedical science and in the delivery of healthcare, and these developments have brought with them important social changes. All too often ethical analysis has lagged behind these changes. The purpose of this series is to provide lively, up-to-date, and authoritative studies for the increasingly large and diverse readership concerned with issues in biomedical ethics—not just healthcare trainees and professionals, but also philosophers, social scientists, lawyers, social workers, and legislators. The series will feature both single-author and multi-author books, short and accessible enough to be widely read, each of them focused on an issue of outstanding current importance and interest. Philosophers, doctors, and lawyers from a number of countries feature among the authors lined up for the series.

Health and the Good Society

Setting Healthcare Ethics in Social Context

ALAN CRIBB

CLARENDON PRESS · OXFORD

OXFORD

UNIVERSITY PRESS

Great Clarendon Street, Oxford OX2 6DP

Oxford University Press is a department of the University of Oxford.
It furthers the University's objective of excellence in research, scholarship,
and education by publishing worldwide in

Oxford New York

Auckland Cape Town Dar es Salaam Hong Kong Karachi
Kuala Lumpur Madrid Melbourne Mexico City Nairobi
New Delhi Shanghai Taipei Toronto

With offices in

Argentina Austria Brazil Chile Czech Republic France Greece
Guatemala Hungary Italy Japan Poland Portugal Singapore
South Korea Switzerland Thailand Turkey Ukraine Vietnam

Oxford is a registered trade mark of Oxford University Press
in the UK and in certain other countries

Published in the United States
by Oxford University Press Inc., New York

© Alan Cribb 2005

British Library Cataloguing in Publication Data
Data available

Library of Congress Cataloging in Publication Data
Data available

Typeset by SPI Publisher Services, Pondicherry, India
Printed in Great Britain
on acid-free paper by
Biddles Ltd, King's Lynn, Norfolk

ISBN 978–0–19–924273–3 (Hbk.)
     978–0–19–923294–9 (Pbk.)

1 3 5 7 9 10 8 6 4 2

Acknowledgements

I would like to thank all my friends and colleagues at King's College London. King's has been a second home to me for almost 15 years and I feel very fortunate to have met and worked with so many wonderful people over that period. I am grateful for the kindness and encouragement of colleagues from the School of Nursing, the Medical School, and the Centre of Medical Law and Ethics. However I owe a special debt to my immediate colleagues in the Centre for Public Policy Research—particularly Stephen Ball, Peter Duncan, Sharon Gewirtz, Meg Maguire, and Deryn Watson—not only for giving me the opportunity to think about and talk about many of the issues in this book, but also for putting up with me on a daily basis. They have all helped me in countless ways. Sharon Gewirtz must be singled out for her special contribution to the production of this book. In some places I draw on work that we have undertaken together. In addition she has read and commented on the chapters, helped me tidy up my thinking, and been a constant source of moral and practical support. Indeed, Sharon took upon herself the responsibility for making sure the text was finished, and I doubt it would have been without her gentle-touch mentoring.

I am very grateful to John Harris and Søren Holm for the invitation to write this book and for involving me in their 'EMPIRE' project (a European Union funded project about the role of empirical research in bioethics)—an involvement which helped me think about the themes I was addressing here. Søren also provided me with some very helpful feedback on an earlier draft. It is 20 years since my first foray into the philosophy and ethics of healthcare, and the conversations I had at that time with David Seedhouse and Harry Lesser (who was the doctoral supervisor to both David and me) have no doubt fed into this work in ways I can no longer trace. More recently George Khushf has been very influential both by example and by providing me with encouragement at those times when I felt I had nothing to say. The fact that people as knowledgeable and talented as these have taken what I have been trying to write about seriously has provided a very real spur. There are many other people in the world of healthcare ethics whose example and friendship have also supported my efforts. I am particularly appreciative of the way I have been 'welcomed back' by UK bioethics colleagues after having spent a long period teaching and writing about other things.

Although this is not the best place to do so I should also say a much deserved thank you to those in my 'first home', i.e. Jacky and the other members of my family. Their love and support are, of course, priceless. Thanks to Jacky, especially, who has had even more to put up with than my immediate colleagues! I hope I can do something worthwhile in return, and I am very clear that writing a book—even one much better than this— does not count.

FOR WILLIAM JOSEPH EDWARD CRIBB—AKA DAD

Preface

Though we suffer and die one by one, both health and healthcare are
social phenomena, whether in those forces that bring poor health or
those that help us overcome it. That it is individuals who have the poor
health and suffer pain that only they can know directly should not
distract our attention from the social contexts and determinants of all
that affects health.

Callahan (1990: 104)

In this book I explore some of the implications of looking at healthcare
ethics in social context. My starting point is the contention that clinical ethics
cannot be insulated from questions in public-health ethics; and the book is in
large part an elaboration and defence of that contention. My purpose is
partly substantive and partly methodological—to ask what happens to 'personal claims' when they are set against 'public claims'; and to see interpersonal healthcare relationships in the context of wider social relations. I hope
that what I have to say will help to reframe some of the problems of
healthcare ethics, and that where I do not attempt solutions this reframing
can be seen as a contribution of its own.

In placing healthcare ethics in social context I am operating with two
rather different but complementary senses of 'the social'. First, I am thinking
about health as a 'social good'. I am interested in the interactions between,
and what I will suggest is, in some respects, a growing convergence between
personal healthcare and public health. This includes the various senses in
which individual health needs to be understood in the context of population
health, and the ways in which professional ethics in healthcare can only be
understood in conjunction with 'institutional ethics' and 'policy ethics'. This
provides the substantive theme of the book.

Second, I am thinking about the 'social construction'[1] of health-related
goods, and acknowledging what might be called the 'sociologizing' of contem-
porary thought. What I mean by 'sociologizing' here can be boiled down to the
widespread recognition of two things: (a) that the categories through which we

---

[1] I am using the expression 'social construction' here, and elsewhere, in a very general sense to
convey the idea of things that are built or created through social and institutional frameworks.
I do not want to ally myself with the quasi-idealistic perspectives in sociology that are often
labelled as 'social constructionism' (Burr, 1995). Of course I accept that 'social things' are partly
constituted by cultures and systems of meaning but there is no sense in which I intend to contrast
what I mean by 'socially constructed' to a realist philosophy of social science.

make sense of health policy and healthcare, including the categories which constitute our own experiences of health and ill-health are not unproblematic, transparent, and neutral tools of representation but are historically and culturally conditioned and value laden; and (b) that what is achieved through our actions is not always fully captured by our immediate, local, or 'first-order' descriptions of them; that social processes can be described from different, including more or less critical, vantage points. Within healthcare the most striking examples of this sociologizing tendency are the manifold challenges to the power of medical science and associated forms of professional authority as the key arbiters of how we should think about, talk about, and act in relation to health. In short, the frameworks of health policy, healthcare, and for that matter healthcare ethics itself are all partly constituted by innumerable implicit value judgements, and can serve to conceal as well as to reveal the nature of social relations. This provides the methodological theme of the book.

The problem set I want to address relates to both of these themes. I want to reframe healthcare ethics as a whole, including clinical ethics, within the broad context of social relations, obligations, and entitlements, and more specifically within the socially embodied 'value field' of health-related action. Although I will sometimes give more emphasis to the first theme (health as a social good) and sometimes more to the second theme (the social construction of health goods) they both need to be considered together, or there is a danger that in questioning the substantive focus of healthcare ethics we will simply assume frameworks and categories relating to health, health professions, or health policy which themselves require questioning. (There is no point arguing that perspective x is better than perspective y for dealing with z but not seeing that z is an inadequate account of the domain.) I have described the second theme as a sociological one in order to acknowledge the substantial contribution of the sociology of health and illness to this area, but—as Peter Winch pointed out almost 50 years ago (Winch, 1958)—there are strong continuities between sociological perspectives and certain currents with the tradition of analytical philosophy. Both sociologists and applied philosophers are interested in unpacking and problematizing received categories, and in certain places I will draw upon both traditions at the same time. Before I offer a summary of the structure and content of the book I will use the example of 'informed consent' to explain and illustrate some of the underlying methodological and substantive concerns which run through the book. First, I want to note the 'slipperiness' of the social world—its context specificity and the contestability of our descriptions of it. Second, I will briefly introduce two of my substantive themes—the relationships between microlevel and macrolevel perspectives, and the possible tensions between the values of 'health' and 'empowerment'.

I think it is important to begin by underlining the contestability of descriptions of the 'social context' of healthcare. Our more confident descriptions of the social world, particularly those descriptions that carve it up into tidy packages, have a misleading aspect. The business of securing informed consent provides a familiar example. How can we decide, in real world settings, whether or not informed consent has been obtained? As an ideal informed consent is relatively clear. But it is notoriously murky in practice. If the principles of informed consent are to have any purchase in the world then the cultures and practices of informed consent have to be *socially and institutionally embodied*; and informed consent has then to be practically *enacted* by specific individuals. Anyone who has taken any interest in this topic will know of cases where informed consent has been 'obtained' in principle but not in practice. This includes cases where institutional procedures have been followed and yet, for one reason or another, the person at the centre of them has been, in some important respects, bypassed. Now this may seem to have more to do with plain bad practice than with the supposed 'slipperiness' of the social world. However I suggest that these factors interrelate and are both important. A conscientious practitioner will be cautious before making claims about 'what is going on' and especially about other people's life-worlds. They will be ready to exercise their 'sociological imagination' as well as their ethical principles.

In practice informed consent can 'fail' for a host of reasons—reasons which relate both to the intrinsic difficulty of making the necessary judgements and to contingencies of specific circumstances. It is not easy to make the judgements about the thresholds of competence, understanding, and voluntariness in general (Beauchamp and Childress, 2001), and it is often difficult to make the practical judgements in particular cases, even given the most conscientious attention to the case and to the individual patient. Such attention merely brings home the compound complexities attaching to the patient and the circumstances of consent. We see, for example, the patient's age, social class, gender, ethnicity, and so on; their level of anxiety or vulnerability; their particular health-related beliefs or personal values; indeed all of the specifics of their identity and subjectivity. Similarly we can pay attention to institutional and professional regimes, procedures, and norms which construct the circumstances of consent and the particular relationships, roles, and actions in play from case to case. As all of these things come into focus so does the precariousness of consent enactments.

This example also allows me to anticipate and briefly illustrate something of the discussion of micro–macro links that runs through the book. In order to improve the quality of informed consent we can pay regard both to particular enactments and to the policies, procedures, and climates of consent. For the former we might ask, 'With what sort of manner, and how skilfully, does this particular health professional tailor her remarks to this particular client; how responsive is she to the client's needs and demands?'

For the latter we might ask, 'How can we create institutional and societal circumstances which foster informed consent, and how can we prepare health professionals and potential patients to make best use of these circumstances? From this we can see that the same participants are engaged in healthcare relationships at a number of levels, including the doctor–patient level and doctor-qua-citizen or patient-qua-citizen level.[2] Ethical analysis of what ought to be done must pay regard to these various levels and the multiple ways in which professional–patient relations and roles are constructed.

To indicate something more about my substantive concerns I want to reflect on the idea of 'creating healthy citizens'. This phrase has been chosen to point to the problematic of public-health policy. It captures the object of public-health policy in a single expression and it also suggests some of the dilemmas facing such policy. These dilemmas can also be approached through the idea of informed consent. The importance of informed consent as a topic in healthcare ethics, and in practice, stems from the way in which it brings together and symbolizes two imperatives of modern health policy. We wish to manage what we hope is the beneficent paternalism of health professionals and also to protect individual autonomy. We wish to harness knowledge to promote health but we also wish to ensure that the intended beneficiaries can participate in decisions about, and processes of, health promotion. These balancing acts between 'well-being' and 'wants' cut through the whole of health policy. There are discourses of quality of life, health promotion, health gain, efficiency, and so on. But these typically interact and, to some degree, compete with other discourses of participation, empowerment, citizenship, and choice.

The fundamental challenge facing the ethics of public-health policy is thus the problem of informed consent writ large. In a modern health polity it is not enough to aim for *healthy* populations—we need to aim for healthy *citizens*. How can we promote health in a way that not only respects autonomy but also builds partnerships for health? And how can we manage the tensions between the values of health and 'empowerment', in both clinical care and public-health policy more generally? These broad questions provide the backcloth to this book, but I am particularly interested in the interactions between clinical healthcare and public-health policy, between the micro- and macro-worlds of healthcare.

---

[2] For the purposes of this book I am taking the level of citizenship within a specific health polity as the most general interpretation of the social context, i.e. I am deliberately, and to some extent arbitrarily, confining myself to the context of national and not international health policy. I must acknowledge that in some respects this is perverse because the most substantively important issues in healthcare ethics are arguably about the global distribution of benefits and burdens. However, these issues are beyond the substantive scope of this book which is predominantly about the relationship between 'professional–client' and 'policy–citizen' perspectives. I will, however, return briefly to the global dimension in the concluding chapter.

The Structure of the Book

The book is divided into four parts. Part 1 (Chapters 1 to 3) expands on this preface by exploring the background to my concerns—which I label 'the diffusion of the health agenda'—and by setting out in much more depth the implications of the changes to the value field of healthcare which result from the opening up of conceptions of health and from greater public involvement in healthcare. Part 2 (Chapters 4 to 6) reviews some overarching questions in health-policy ethics. It looks in particular at questions relating to health promotion, inequalities in health, and personal responsibility for health. Part 3 (Chapters 7 to 9) considers related changes to the landscape of healthcare professional ethics. How is professional ethics influenced by changes in the social and policy landscape including the rise in managerialism and reforming discourses represented by health promotion? Part 4 (Chapters 10 to 12) returns to issues about health-policy agenda setting and healthcare ethics. How can education support public inclusion in health-policy debate, and what should such debate be about? Finally, what are the implications of the book for health education and healthcare ethics?

As noted above, one of my starting points is the claim that the micro- and macro-worlds of healthcare are, to put it boldly, *in fact* merging into one another. (A claim I will return to in a more measured way as I proceed.) I begin to illustrate the thinking behind this claim in Chapter 1. There I introduce the 'diffusion of the health agenda'—the many ways in which health-related debates and practices have 'opened up' to include more and more elements, and 'wider' and 'deeper' perspectives relating, for example, to health determinants or psychosocial factors. This diffusion, I argue, is closely connected to very broad sets of social changes which cluster around the rise in 'social reflexivity', i.e. a pervasive and growing self-consciousness about the social construction of our health experiences and practices. The rise in social reflexivity, I suggest, has major implications for the focus and methodology of healthcare ethics as a discipline. Namely, that it needs to orient itself more around the two themes I have already introduced: health as a social good and the social construction of health goods.

One of the ways in which broader social agendas are 'carried into' health policies and practices are by some of the 'reforming' discourses I have already mentioned, such as those of evidence-based healthcare, person-centred healthcare, and health promotion. Through discursive shifts the, sometimes competing, clusters of goods that these reforms represent are both intentionally and unintentionally built into the value field of healthcare. The topics of Chapters 2 and 3 are chosen to illustrate the diffused agenda more fully, and relate to the two health-policy imperatives discussed above.

These are arguably the two most powerful discursive currents in recent health policy: the drive to optimize the effectiveness of interventions to produce the most or best 'health outcomes', and the push towards higher levels of 'lay involvement' in healthcare and health policy. In both chapters I take these different, and sometimes competing, currents seriously on their own terms but also critically examine their ethical significance. In particular in Chapter 2 I try to set 'health outcomes' in the context of the other, and 'thicker', individual and social goods represented by a more diffused agenda; and in Chapter 3 I question the extent to which wider participation can be justified in practice, and also highlight some of the tensions between participation in care and participation in policy. Using these themes I also begin to illustrate what I mean by the value field of health, including the structures, cultures, and institutional frameworks which shape conduct and help to create the 'ethical spaces' through which roles and obligations are defined.

In Chapters 4, 5, and 6 I debate a number of questions in public-health policy ethics, beginning in Chapter 4 with a consideration of the nature and ethics of health promotion. Health promotion is used here, and elsewhere in the book, to represent the reforming discourses of the diffused health agenda. It is a movement which attempts to encapsulate many of the 'enlarged' concerns of modern healthcare—a bigger time–space orientation, a population orientation, and a 'positive health' or well-being orientation. In Chapter 4 I examine the ways in which health promotion amounts to a new set of problems for healthcare ethics. I use health promotion to illustrate the social construction of 'healthcare', as a particular social and ethical constellation, and to illustrate the interactions between clinical ethics and social ethics, and thus the need to consider health professional ethics at the macro- as well as the micro-level.

In Chapter 5 and 6 I continue the argument for this multilevel analysis in healthcare ethics but do so through discussing the substantive theme of the social distribution of health-related goods and obligatons. Chapter 5 focuses specifically on health inequalities. What is the ethical significance of health inequalities and can we make sense of a collective obligation, arising from a commitment to some conception of social justice, to attempt to rectify such inequalities? I argue in favour of such a putative obligation whilst stressing the many challenges which threaten to undercut, or dissolve, its import. Although I concentrate upon the importance of tackling the 'social class gradient' in mortality and morbidity I also set out the need to interpret the challenge of health inequalities more broadly, as involving a range of axes in which we are all implicated. Chapter 6 maintains this theme and argues for a diffused responsibility for the directions and outcomes of health policy, including health inequalities. It also explores the ways in which such responsibilities have to be, to some degree, socially defined and established—our responsibilities cannot be identified in complete abstraction from the social definition of our roles and mutual expectations. I argue that specific questions about healthcare entitlements and obligations have to be answered in the context of a broader societal analysis of these things, and of the ways in which responsibilities are realized in institutional and policy frameworks.

In Chapters 7, 8, and 9 the focus is directly on setting professional ethics in the context of institutional norms and social policies. Given the preceding analysis of policy ethics and the related accounts of how the value field of healthcare is changing in the light of many discursive shifts, what are the implications for professional ethics? Chapter 7 introduces the themes and arguments of this part of the book. It examines the social construction of professional roles and the relationships between what I call 'vocational' and 'institutional' identities. It thereby illustrates and begins to investigate the division of ethical labour in healthcare. Chapter 8 looks at the role of healthcare management both as an important form of healthcare agency in its own right and as a set of discourses and mechanisms which mediate between the policy context and institutional and professional practices. How, it asks, does management reconstruct professional subjectivities and healthcare goods? In particular I question the extent to which professional practice is being, and ought to be, reoriented around various social agendas including, but not only, public health ends. Chapter 9 pursues this issue further by concentrating on the revisions to professional roles and identities represented by health promotion. How do these and analogous revisions change the nature and legitimacy of professional–client relationships, and what would be the basis for resisting or welcoming these changes? It considers the tensions inherent in the reconstruction of professional roles, and thereby also further illustrates the need for healthcare ethics to work at the level of role construction as well as at the level of action. Together these three chapters press home the question of how health policy can achieve a balance between personal and social agendas in general, and between person-centred care and population-oriented policy in particular.

Chapter 10 sets out to review the potential role of health education in supporting a more informed and 'empowered' public involvement in deliberation about health-related decision-making. It argues that a diffused health agenda presents new educational challenges and opportunities, and it reviews some of the dilemmas that confront such a reimagined health education. In particular it considers the tensions between education as a health technology and education as social and political empowerment, and argues that there is no easy resolution of these tensions. Chapters 11 and 12 review the main arguments and implications of the book, Chapter 11 exploring the methodological and Chapter 12 the substantive implications of my arguments. They summarize the case for a socially reflexive healthcare ethics, arguing that both action and the value field of action should form the subject matter of healthcare ethics, and they illustrate some of the key debates facing public-health policy. The value field of healthcare is presented as something that is both 'caused' and chosen. In other words as something that has to be understood, in part, sociologically but also as something to be approached, debated and shaped with ethical purpose.

Contents

PART I

The Evolving Value Field of Healthcare

1

Introduction: The Diffusion of the Health Agenda

This chapter explains the 'diffusion of the health agenda', and its implications for healthcare and healthcare ethics. Chapters 2 and 3 extend this account of the diffused agenda by debating two of its most important dimensions: the opening up of the 'ends' of health policy, and the opening up of levels of 'involvement' in healthcare and policy. I will begin with a thumbnail sketch of some fundamental shifts in modern health policy and services, and then look briefly at some of the philosophical changes that underpin these shifts, in particular what I will call 'the social turn' in healthcare. In the second half of the chapter I reflect upon some of the implications of this diffused agenda for healthcare ethics.

Sarah Nettleton (1995: 12) has usefully set out what she calls 'a crude indication of a range of transformations' taking place within healthcare (see Fig.1). Each pair of terms is used to indicate a whole complex of shifts in emphasis and orientation that have and are taking place in health policy.

Here I am not so much interested in this sketch as history, in assessing the validity, sensitivity and explanation of these shifts, as in their implications for understanding healthcare. But it is worth noting that these transformations arise out of a compound of economic, epidemiological, and cultural factors. They reflect 'real' changes in patterns of mortality and morbidity in the rich countries of the world as well as those embodied in such things as the rise of

Disease	Health
Hospital	Community
Acute	Chronic
Cure	Prevention
Intervention	Monitoring
Treatment	Care
Patient	Person

Fig. 1. *'Diffusion' of the Health Agenda.*

consumerism. Theories of 'health transition', as well as their limitations, are much debated in the public-health literature (Beaglehole and Bonita, 1997) but the rise during the twentieth century in the relative importance of non-communicable diseases such as heart disease, stroke, and the cancers is well documented, as is the problem of people living longer but often living with chronic illness of one sort or another. Different problems demand different solutions and healthcare has naturally turned to an array of environmental and educational approaches. Educational approaches—if education is properly understood—necessitate working 'with' people and not just 'on' them, and the same can be said about any environmental or public-policy strategy in a democratic context.

Figure 1 serves as an illustration of the 'diffusion' of the health agenda. The terms in the second column are more open-ended than those in the first. They refer to things that are more spread out in time and space and/ or are more multifaceted. Generally speaking they imply the need for partnerships rather than for circumscribed technical interventions.

What do I mean by the diffusion of the health agenda? Roughly speaking I am taking 'the health agenda' to refer to the ways in which health is 'talked about', and thus acted on, in society, including both *what* is on the agenda, and *who* sets the agenda. It is shorthand for a range of considerations. Likewise the phrase 'the diffusion of the health agenda' has been coined as shorthand for a cluster of shifts and transformations such as those indicated above. By the use of a single phrase I do not want to imply that there is one essential underlying process which provides coherence to this cluster. On the contrary these shifts are, in many respects, in tension with one another, but the idea of 'diffusion' does suggest what seems to me to be a useful generalization—that the health agenda is, at least in some important ways, becoming more dispersed.[1]

For a snapshot of what is meant by diffusion we can contrast a routine hospital operation with a typical national healthy-eating campaign. At least at first sight the differences are substantial. The former can be seen as a relatively closed system—it takes place in a confined time and space, both its ends and the procedures it involves can, by and large, be specified in technical terms, and it is fairly well insulated from other aspects of life. The latter can be seen as a relatively open system—it takes place over a long period and in many different settings and spaces, its ends and methods are typically contested, and it intersects with a host of other public policy and private considerations.

---

[1] There are arguably other countervailing forces—centrefugal rather than centrepetal ones— the discussion later in the book (in Part 3) of managerialism and the population-oriented values which tend to underpin it, provides a crucial example.

Of course these distinctions are exaggerated, and are partly a matter of appearance rather than substance, but they are central to understanding and appraising a range of influential currents in healthcare. These currents, including an increasing emphasis on prevention, on health inequalities, on the management of chronic illness, and on lay participation in healthcare, are commonly discussed under the umbrella of challenges to the 'medical model'. Up to a point this is a useful story, and the medical model is a useful idealization, but the full story is much less tidy. I will not pretend to tell that story here but simply note that medicine has always had holistic aspects, has been formed through internal debate as well as external critique, and has evolved through a number of diverse historical forms. The recent history of changes to the health agenda can be written either as an account of the displacement of medicine or as part of the history of medicine, albeit with a different orientation and with a different stress. But however it is written it has involved a growing recognition of the importance of the social context of health and healthcare. This growing recognition is produced not only by the influence of sociology, and other social sciences, in healthcare but also by the rise of what might be seen as 'a sociological attitude' across society—what is sometimes called 'social reflexivity' (Giddens, 1991).

The Social Turn—Towards an Understanding of the Diffusion

I will not pretend to offer an explanation for the whole cluster of shifts which I am labelling as the diffusion of the health agenda but I think it is worth saying something more about its close interrelationship with the 'social turn' in healthcare.

The social turn is made up of many elements which are manifest in the diffusion of the health agenda. I will just say a little about what might be seen as the three fundamental elements of the turn, i.e. an increased emphasis upon: (a) the social environment, (b) subjectivity and the interpersonal, and (c) social reflexivity. These three elements occur in different forms and combinations, and it is their combined effects which are the most powerful; but they can be presented separately:

(a) The social environment, by definition, encompasses so much. Even if we exclude the material environment (which would be odd because society interpenetrates the physical world) we can think about the causes of health in terms of, for example, social structures, social groups, policies and institutions, cultures and norms. And within 'the social' we can include economic, political, and religious aspects, etc. Different social scientists emphasize different items on these lists and employ different paradigms but, whatever their approach, their work not only illuminates the causes of ill-health but also what Callahan, as cited at the beginning of the Preface, calls the forces 'that help us overcome' ill-health, i.e. the full panoply of public policies, health professions, and healthcare. Those involved in healthcare are increasingly preoccupied with understanding whether and how 'it works' and what other effects it has; whether they seek this understanding in the language of health economics, medical anthropology, or evidence-based medicine.

(b) Subjectivity and the interpersonal—the social certainly includes the cultural—the world of meanings and persons (as opposed to bodies), and we now understand a great deal more about the crucial causal and constitutive roles of culture and individual subjectivity in health and well-being. Healthcare is widely understood to be both a 'technical' and an interpersonal enterprise; one which has to take account of both cultural factors in general and, more particularly, the perspectives and points of view of individuals. Health professionals, in many settings and instances, are, for example, expected to consider the meaning and self-understanding of illness experiences; and perhaps to actively engage in the construction of meaning and narrative, such as in 'therapeutic emplotment' (Del Vecchio Good *et al.*, 1994). It is in this area where medical humanities play such an important role by furnishing insight into human life-worlds and their construction.

(c) Social reflexivity: social reflexivity is now a commonplace phenomenon. Its nature, importance, and relevance for healthcare ethics will be elaborated further in the next section. In modern health polities it is quite normal for people to understand themselves as products of their specific historical circumstances, and the mass media continuously bolster this form of self-consciousness by reporting and dissecting research into the 'social causes' of our experiences, including our health experiences. Hence, whether or not we think that medicine has been displaced somewhat from the centre of gravity of healthcare it has certainly been placed in context. First, there is a widespread understanding that there are many other determinants of health than the work of doctors or other health professionals. Secondly, the organization of health services and the regulation of health professionals are themselves considered to be a matter for public debate. Thus the structures and cultures of healthcare are increasingly experienced as historically contingent, and are to some degree subject to public choice.

Daniel Callahan is not alone in drawing our attention to 'the social contexts and determinants of all that affects health'. There is now an established role for a wide range of social sciences and humanities in healthcare and medical education. Indeed, the challenge that social sciences and humanities pose for healthcare is no longer one of mere 'acceptance' but rather the challenges raised by the potential proliferation of social-science related disciplines and subdisciplines.

The combined effects of the three elements of the social turn reviewed above are profound. It is not just that the agenda of health professionals is more diffuse, encompassing myriad social concerns and individual perspectives, it is also that the content of the 'health agenda' is no longer the preserve of health professionals. The making of the health agenda is itself diffused (and debated) across society. Health professionals have to negotiate their place, roles, and relations in the public space of policy-makers, managers, and clients.

There is yet another sense in which the social turn contributes to the diffusion of the health agenda. Diffusion is not only manifested in *what* is on the agenda, and *who* makes the agenda; it is also manifested in the intrinsic *indeterminacy* of the agenda. Social understanding is inherently plural and contested. There is comparatively little closure in the social sciences—once we place politics, culture, and individual subjectivity on the health agenda we have to be prepared to live with compound forms of debate and uncertainty. We may not wish to go all the way with the more zealous advocates of 'post-modern' scepticism and abandon truth claims for permanent deconstruction, but we have to move into a world of competing 'readings' and authorities. This is a world in which the continuing authority of clinical science is no longer guaranteed by its would-be foundational credentials but has to be earned in the market place of ideas and concerns. A world in which, to take an extreme but pertinent example, some doctors find themselves at public inquiries subject to the critical gaze of health-policy experts, ethicists, the media, the public, and their patients. A world in which superficially neutral concepts such as 'what is medically indicated' or 'what is medically necessary' have become problematized as obfuscations of necessarily value-laden judgement (Dickenson, 1999).

Just as doctors are learning to see their patients in social context, the world has also learned to see doctors in social context. Doctors look through the social lens and see everyone else looking back at them, and making their own diagnoses. It is often said that these days doctors have to be prepared to deal with patients who have access to all kinds of knowledge about their clinical conditions and treatments. That is the least of it. These days a doctor may be expected to engage in balancing clinical judgements, budget judgements, emotional judgements, and policy judgements, *and* deal with patients, managers, and policy-makers who, in many cases, understand that all of this is going on. Furthermore each of these parties might have their own views about how these various balancing acts should best be executed, and how the organization of healthcare might be improved to this end.

To return to Nettleton's helpful figure (Fig. 1), it is not that there has been some absolute shift away from the things in the left-hand column and towards those things on the right. It would be bizarre to claim that diseases, patients, and hospitals are somehow becoming less significant. Rather what is happening is that the left-hand items are more typically, more routinely, being seen *in the context* of the right-hand items. These shifts take place within a number of different paradigms but what they all bring is a wider and deeper frame of reference for healthcare. To conclude I will stress just three aspects of the emerging frame of reference. First, it means that the whole of the world is opened up as a potential site of healthcare intervention. Second, it means seeing personal health in the context of public health, and thereby raises questions about the relationship between health as a personal good and health as a public good. Third, it means seeing the language, and the authority of, clinical science in the context of a complex web of overlapping, competing, and more conspicuously value-laden social judgements. Social reflexivity is thus both a cause and consequence of the diffusion of the health agenda.

Social Reflexivity and Healthcare Ethics

Some discussions of healthcare ethics begin by exploring technological change, and the ways in which new technologies challenge our categories and pose novel philosophical and ethical puzzles. I have chosen to concentrate on a related, but arguably more fundamental, aspect of late modernity—the way in which social reflexivity reframes the health agenda. One way of characterizing social reflexivity is to see it as the incorporation of a kind of sociological mind-set into everyday life. Giddens defines what he calls 'institutional reflexivity' as 'the regularised use of knowledge about circumstances of social life as a constitutive element in its organisation and transformation' (1991: 20). For present purposes a paradigm example of institutional reflexivity is health-service management (and for that reason I will return to it in several places). Management is about using information about services to change services and, of course, the presence of management systems itself changes services. Providing services under the gaze of managers means somehow 'taking into account' the goals and norms of institutional management. It creates new climates and relations.

But, of course, reflexivity does not only apply to the making and remaking of institutions, it applies to all aspects of social and personal life. For example, as Giddens points out, people who get divorced and remarried now may do so informed by countless pieces of journalistic and academic research and analysis into changing relationship patterns, the potential effects of divorce, ways of coping, and so on. This level of social self-consciousness does not only 'report' changes it partly constitutes them. Social understanding creates new social realities.

All of this applies as much to healthcare values as it does to health. Just as we can now investigate the ways in which social and institutional structures and discourses produce health, we can investigate the ways in which they produce the 'value field' of healthcare. In neither case can we afford simply to concentrate on the intentions and actions of health professionals and policy-makers. As was briefly illustrated in the Preface in relation to informed consent we need to look not only at the intentions and self-understanding of the actors but also at the pressures, norms, climates, and cultures that shape understanding and actions. The salience attached to consent within a particular setting, tacit evaluations of the role and relative importance of consent, and the ways in which consent procedures are interpreted and enacted are all shaped both by individual choices and by the value field in which the choices are made.

Indeed to put it in this way—to distinguish between actor and context—is in some ways misleading. It might create the impression of two essentially independent things 'bumping into' one another. The crux of the sociological mind-set is the recognition that the actor and the social field interpenetrate one another and are mutually constitutive. Different sociologists express this idea within different theoretical frameworks, and hence with different terms and emphases, but something like this idea is an inescapable feature of social reflexivity. Giddens, for example, has elaborated this idea within what he terms 'structuration theory'—an attempt to combine structure and agency in sociological explanation. He writes, 'In and through their activities agents reproduce the conditions that make these activities possible' (Giddens 1984: 2). Social constraints and cultures are partly created by individuals and in turn these constraints and cultures shape the possibilities of individual action.

This has substantial implications for the focus and conduct of healthcare ethics. It means that healthcare ethics has to consider the actor's social field in conjunction with the actor's reasoning and choice making. For purposes of illustration I will stick with the example of informed consent: imagine health professional A and patient B. Assuming that what we are interested in, for now, is B's interests and well-being then it is no good simply examining A's understanding of and commitment to the principles of informed consent. What we need to consider are the ways in which the whole setting and the conditions of interaction (including, of course, the thoughts and actions of the individuals involved) support, undermine, or refract the enactment of consent. Looking across a range of settings we might, for example, question why consent is interpreted fairly minimally in some but more fully in others. Why, for example, is the prescription of drugs sometimes done with a 'lighter touch' consent process than surgical intervention? Or, to take another kind of example, why might those working on one hospital ward seem to place much more emphasis on professional–patient communication (including the ensuring of consent where appropriate) than those on another ward in the same hospital? Some of the time there may be good reasons for these differences and the settings, and thinking within them, may embody these good reasons. But often we will have to turn to more contingent 'causes' such as professional traditions and distinctive institutional norms and subcultures for an explanation. We would need a model such as that of structuration theory to support our explanations, a model which sees individual choices as both shaping, and as shaped by, the social context. If we care about B's interests and well-being then we have to take as much interest in the way values are embodied in the social field of health as we do in the principles of consent and A's understanding of them.

Paying due attention to the social context of health, and specifically to the value field of health-related action, means that healthcare ethics needs to be genuinely interdisciplinary. It has not only to draw upon philosophical ethics and law but also find ways of properly integrating these with historical and social science perspectives. One part of this is to recognize the contribution that empirical research can make to the domain of healthcare ethics, and in particular to see that this is not just about gathering 'the facts' for the ethicist's mill but it is about understanding how ethics is so-to-speak socially created, an understanding which requires social as well as philosophical theory.

In what I have said so far about the importance of the social field I have relied on crude distinctions between constraints and cultures, or more generally still, between structures and discourses. The rationale for making these kinds of distinctions is to point towards the many different ways in which social contexts shape actions and experiences—ways which are more or less overt, more or less voluntaristic, and more or less rational. I may do something, for example, because I am instructed by my employer to do it, or because I am more or less conscious of the incentives and disincentives that attach to it. Or I may do something because the contexts which shape my role have sets of assumptions and values built into them which, to put it crudely, 'colonize' my thoughts and actions. In the latter case I am not calculatively taking into account the overt institutional pressures and norms, I am acting spontaneously on the basis of values which are ingrained in my working agendas and practices.

Whether we talk about structural causes of action or the discursive construction of action depends upon what phenomena we are describing but it also depends to some extent, of course, on how we theorize the social field. (I will not review these differences here but there are, for example, more materialist and more idealist theories, and there are also more or less comprehensive conceptions of 'discourse'.) The different forms of social influence, crudely summarized above, are closely related to the distinction which Foucault makes between 'sovereign' and 'disciplinary' forms of power. The former is the overt and official power of 'governors' (broadly understood) to determine the options and actions of 'the governed', the latter is not confined to the formally powerful, nor deliberately exercised, rather it is discursively accomplished and diffused, with the lines of force flowing in multiple directions. Disciplinary power can be seen, to oversimplify, in how 'the way we do things here' influences the things each of us does. Foucault directs our attention to 'the manifold relationships of force that take shape and come into play in the machinery of production, in families, in limited groups, and institutions' (Foucault, 1978: 94).

What I am arguing is that healthcare ethics has to incorporate an interest in the value field of health policy and healthcare, in the processes that construct this value field, and in the construction of ethics by this value field. What I have called the diffusion of the health agenda can be understood as the incorporation of many emerging discourses—often competing discourses—into the arena of health. There are increasingly influential discourses of public health and health promotion, around, for example, priority setting, prevention, empowerment, partnership, health inequalities, etc. There are also overlapping multiple discourses of biomedical reform, around, for example, priority setting, health promotion, person-centredness, and evidenced-based healthcare. These discourses, considered individually and in complex networks, bring about changes to the value field of health-related action, and construct 'ethical possibilities' within specific settings. In short, the shifts in health policy that I sketched earlier do not only construct different health agendas they construct different ethical agendas. I will return to this notion later in this chapter and throughout the book.

Social reflexivity, therefore, makes possible and demands new *approaches* in healthcare ethics, but the 'social turn' in health policy also precipitates new *substantive* ethical questions. Healthcare is itself increasingly constituted by the social sciences and social reflexivity. The increased understanding of subjectivity and the 'social meanings' constitutive of health and healthcare experiences represents one set of revisions which 'deepen' the medical frame of reference to—broadly speaking—include subjectivity and culture as well as biology. The increased understanding of the social determinants of health and disease represent another set of revisions which 'widen' the medical frame of reference to include all aspects of the natural and social world as potential points of intervention. The former entails supplementing the focus on disease management. The latter entails, in addition, the possibility of managing the causes of disease and not merely its expression. (These two tendencies interact in complex ways which cannot be fully rehearsed here; however it should be clear that they are in some ways in tension with one another, the former potentially qualifying the importance of biomedical approaches, the latter potentially extending their influence.) These 'deepening' and 'widening' aspects of the diffusion introduce new dimensions to ethical debates about the 'ends' and means' of healthcare. What ought healthcare to aim at, and how can various health-related goods be weighed together? And what kinds of interventions in our physical and social environment can be legitimated in the name of health?

These are questions I will return to in the next few chapters. However, even to state these questions in this general form illustrates the substantive implications of the diffusion for healthcare ethics. When health and disease are seen as essentially social phenomena, when we speak of them in the language either of culture or social determinants, we are, to some extent, bound to frame the practical debate of what to do about them with reference to social ends. If my experience of illness is partly constituted by socio-cultural stigmas, or if my illness could most easily have been prevented by putting something in the water supply, then we are forced to think about 'social solutions', I cannot be 'treated' purely on my own. In these sorts of cases it is not possible to insulate the ethics of my treatment from the wider ethical field or from debates about social goods or values.

Now one way of capturing these points is to shift the focus from clinical ethics to what might be called public-health ethics. The latter, it could be said, is roughly the set of ethical issues which has arisen from the diffusion of the health agenda. It is necessarily concerned with social ends and it does call for a rather different style of healthcare ethics which is complementary to the more narrowly focused concerns of clinical ethics. Other commentators have made related points by criticizing the inherent 'myopia' of much traditional medical ethics which concentrates too much on the near to hand rather than the underlying social processes and context (or, a closely related concern, which takes for granted specific institutional or national contexts (Campbell, 2000)). This account is, I believe, broadly correct. But I also want to question the idea that there is a clear distinction to be made between public-health ethics and clinical ethics, and that the former is merely complementary to the latter. This idea seems to me to rest upon a kind of 'innocence' which is no longer sustainable precisely because of the processes of diffusion described above. Just as I have argued that clinical phenomena need to be understood in the context of social phenomena, then clinical ethics has to be addressed in the context of public-health ethics. The widespread penetration of institutional and social reflexivity mean that all healthcare relationships are now routinely seen as, and shaped as, elements in wider social systems. The most conspicuous examples of this shift are the discourses listed above (health promotion, priority setting, etc.) through which healthcare is increasingly often conceived, regulated, and managed. These discourses, in different ways², have public policy ends, and often 'social agendas', built into them, and these ends and related values are, in turn, embodied in the healthcare structures and cultures produced by them. This is what I meant earlier by the bold claim that the micro- and macro-worlds of healthcare are, in some respects, merging. My suggestion here is that (something like) 'public health values' are increasingly shaping not only the general health agenda but also the mundane experiences of face-to-face healthcare.

Thus a socially reflexive healthcare ethics is, in many respects, a public-health ethics (I explore this idea more fully in Chapter 11.) But this is not only a question of scope. As I have noted the emphasis on the value field of health-related action raises questions about appropriate methods in healthcare ethics—with greater salience given to the kinds of methods needed to explore social contexts—but also raises questions about forms of reasoning in health-care and healthcare ethics. It is not merely that the diffused agenda highlights the social construction of the choices that we can make, it is also that, as I have indicated, it highlights the inherent contestability of the value field and the many competing voices that have a stake in it. What I have been talking about adds up, in many respects, to a move away from the positivist outlook of much biomedicine. This means giving up some of the temptations and simplifications of a more technological, instrumental, and value-neutral model of reasoning, a move from a kind of technicism towards a fuller acknowledgement of value contests. For many this signifies a threat. How can this move be achieved without a slide into relativism or subjectivism, without abandoning the possibility of rigour, of some claim to rationality? I want to suggest that this move away from technicism in healthcare not only fails to undercut the potential of deliberative healthcare ethics but rather it moves healthcare ethics, as a mode of deliberation, to the core of health-related decision-making. In the remainder of the chapter I will elucidate the significance of this move from technicism to social and ethical reflexivity in more depth, and in so doing defend the relevance of social reflexivity to a deliberative healthcare ethics.

Technicism and Incommensurability in Health Policy

The growth of interest in questions about the distribution of health-related goods symbolizes the changes I have been reviewing. Debates about

---

² This is an important qualification, although some of these discourses (e.g. 'tackling inequalities') seem to strongly reflect a conception of the public good, with others (e.g. 'person-centredness') any such conception is, at most, only implicit. In these instances, for example, the first case encompasses distributive and/ or 'relational' conceptions within the public good, whereas the second case may simply be pointing to what is valuable to each person (and thus to all people).

inequalities in health, equity of access, and resource allocation or priority setting are characteristic of the diffusion of the health agenda and of the growing influence of public-health agendas. As we bring the social context of health into view we inevitably raise questions about patterns of health and illness and patterns of provision. There is an immediate link in logic between the epidemiologist asking questions about causes of incidence and prevalence and the public-health preoccupation with inequalities in health. It is now well established that one of the major causes of inequalities in mortality and morbidity are underlying inequalities in wealth and life chances. Furthermore even within modern health polities there are well-known differentials in access to healthcare with, for example, more than 40 million US citizens lacking health insurance. And it is a comparatively short step to ask whether, and what, measures ought to be taken to rectify some of these inequalities in health experiences and in access, or to other debates about distributive justice in health and healthcare.

But questions of distribution or 'resource allocation' are notoriously difficult, not least because all health policy entails weighing competing goods. We want to create a healthier society but, as I have stressed, that typically means promoting health in a way that is compatible with respecting people's choices. People value many other things in addition to health and, of course, there are different conceptions of, and dimensions of, health itself. So, how should we manage these balancing acts? How, even in principle, can policy-makers balance, for example, care and cure, or length of life and quality of life? Or how can they balance those things which matter specifically to individuals and those that have a broader social relevance? The problem is, of course, that these goods are of different kinds. There is no obvious 'common denominator' which would enable us to make quantitative comparisons between them. They are, at least in that respect, incommensurable. And even if we could find ways of balancing health-related goals the problem of incommensurability reasserts itself when it comes to balancing health against other goods, or balancing the interests of individuals against those of the population as a whole.

It is important to highlight the problem of incommensurability because there are powerful currents in health policy which serve to disguise it. Both an informal and a formal reductionism often enter the language. The very fact that we speak of health policy or health promotion 'in a single breath' can suggest that we are talking about one thing. This thing, 'health', is surely a good thing so 'more' of it is better than 'less'. Health policy-makers must therefore find the most effective means of creating more of it. On reflection we can see that each of these steps is misleading and contestable, but unexamined these steps exert a plausible and powerful influence. More formally these manoeuvres are built into the preoccupation with effectiveness, efficiency, and evidence-based healthcare. Although there is clearly an important role for examining 'what works' including questions of cost-effectiveness it is essential to be wary of any gloss of value-neutrality which might be associated with these things. For any measure of effectiveness we can always ask (a) what values are built into this model of effectiveness, and (b) how effective, in this respect, do we wish to be, i.e. what other valuable things will be sacrificed in pursuing this conception of effectiveness? The technicism, and the accompanying forms of reductionism, that have the effect of obscuring these questions, are a profoundly important element of the construction of the value field of healthcare. Technicism is deeply embedded in healthcare-policy discourses (and I explore this importance in other places in the book, in particular in Chapter 8 in relation to evidence-based healthcare). And it is not simply a matter of unarticulated reductionism. Sometimes measures of effectiveness are also explicit technical attempts to 'solve' (aspects of) the problem of incommensurability. The most famous example here being that of Quality-adjusted life years (QALYs), which are designed to achieve quantitative comparison between, and aggregation of, the effects of qualitatively different health interventions. QALYs have come to prominence as part of the ever more insistent resource allocation debates. Although there is no apparent common denominator between quality of life and length of life QALYs are an attempt to invent one by combining these two 'outputs' of healthcare into a single measure. And although different healthcare interventions aim at rather different things they might all be said to aim at producing QALYs. Hence the language of QALYs seems to offer an increase in commensurability. I discuss the nature of health-related goods further in Chapter 2; here I am simply noting those movements in policy that serve to disguise the inherent normativity of all our goals and conceptions of success. The development of quantitative measurements fosters a sense of value neutrality which cannot survive inspection.

Whatever the potential usefulness of quantitative measures such as these in managing the problem of incommensurability, they do not even touch some of the deepest problems of resource allocation. At base resource allocation in healthcare is not about 'what is the comparative value of different "health outputs"?' but rather about 'who gets what?' Even if we could straightforwardly answer the former question this does not provide us with any allocative principles. We have to decide independently whether 'valuable outputs' should go, for example, to those who pay for them, those who deserve them, or those who need them (leaving aside the issue of interpreting and operationalizing these things). Obviously policies and practices cannot embody every principle at once. They cannot even embody both 'efficiency' and 'equity', except in some qualified sense in which the two are somehow balanced together. Here again we will find ourselves struggling with different competing goods and systems of value which have to be directly addressed. Masking these contests with technicalities does not help.

Efficiency and equity provide a familiar example of the fundamental goods at stake in health-policy making and of the influence of public-health values on health policy. This is obvious in the case of equity which is overtly a social good. The concept of efficiency may be applied to a single intervention on a single individual but, in the main, the concept has force because there is a need to ensure that resources within a system or scheme are 'stewarded' effectively. Effective stewardship might just mean using resources for the collective good of the relevant tax-payers or scheme contributors. Alternatively some might argue that it demands using resources to advance the collective good of populations irrespective of contributions. In either case both equity and efficiency can be cited as reasons to limit the resources— money, time, scarce technology—devoted to any individual claim. Individuals, and their doctors, are increasingly having to come to terms with not necessarily getting what they judge they need or deserve because of conflicting population claims. These tensions between individual and population claims upon healthcare resources, and between different dimensions of population claims, are cited here as the best-known example of the influence of 'public-health values' on clinical care. They are merely one illustration of the value contests inherent in all policy deliberation; value contests which defy purely technicist solutions. It is important to see that although these contests will sometimes give rise to overt 'dilemmas'—where a health professional has, for example, to explain to an individual how and why she is managing her budget—in the main these tensions are played out less overtly through the construction of the social field of action, for example, in institutional parameters and protocols. Different constructs of 'what matters' in health policy are embedded in the organization and discourses of healthcare. One of the tasks of healthcare ethics must be to unpack and analyse the ways in which different value sets are socially embodied and the many value contests which are played out overtly or covertly. This means uncovering the limitations of technicist models and decision-making approaches. But this task—setting out inherent value contests and the ways in which they are often masked—cannot be the only function of healthcare ethics. What about, for example, the aspiration to offer better solutions to these contests?

Reason and Culture

I have tended to write about the issues of healthcare ethics as essentially practical ones. How, I have asked, might policy-makers, or others, make choices about them? But they are also, to some degree, questions we want to be able to approach using the resources of reason, including the many theoretical resources we have available to help formulate, analyse, and answer them. What is more, the practice of health-policy debate (as of public discourse generally) assumes that the quality of our answers will depend upon us being able to articulate defensible reasons and arguments in their support. Thus we would be foolish to ignore the tradition of work on these and related questions in applied philosophy and analytic healthcare ethics. At the very least this work can provide practical men and women, policy-makers, and citizens, with some theoretical tools, conceptual clarification and argumentative templates with which to analyse and debate policy controversies.

For these reasons I am confident that analytic healthcare ethics can support deliberations about these practical questions. But I cannot leave it at that. To do so would be to fudge the distinction between different approaches to healthcare ethics and their respective ambitions. To put it starkly, is the role of healthcare ethics to provide some intellectual spring cleaning for policy-makers or is it to enable a critique of the assumptions of health policy? Is it to serve conventional healthcare or to rethink it? This wording exaggerates the choice but makes the point.

Lying behind these different forms of ambition are different analyses of the relationship between theory and practice. One set of issues is pragmatic. What are the real-world mechanisms for academic work in healthcare ethics to influence the practical world of healthcare? But underlying these concerns are a more fundamental set of uncertainties. What is the role of reason in practical affairs, and in particular, how far are forms of practical rationality internal to particular societies, health systems, and institutions? Alternatively can we take seriously the idea of some kind of transcendent form of 'reason' which would enable us to objectively appraise and challenge conventional ethics from a more secure standpoint?[3] Before responding to these questions I want to pull together some of the threads of this introductory chapter.

I have been drawing attention to the 'value field' of healthcare and the social construction of that field. Clinical encounters can only be understood in the context of the institutional frameworks and mechanisms in which they take place, and these institutional regimes can only be understood in the

---

[3] It is now, of course, fashionable to decry notions of a universalist 'Reason', and criticism has been made of the presumption of bioethics, or some bioethics, in this regard. For example Maclean (1993) has criticized bioethics in precisely these terms and sets this abstract rationalism against a more Wittgensteinian conception of bioethics as exploring and unpacking values and obligations within cultural and institutional traditions. I cannot explore these fundamental epistemological questions here, but I am not convinced that we have to choose between 'Reason' and 'Culture'. Practical reason is embedded in both cultural traditions and cultural critique, and is not merely internal to cultural forms.

context of the health system and health-policy complex of which they are a part. Value judgements of many different kinds are inevitably built into these systems and institutional regimes. These judgements are more or less overt and are made more or less deliberately. The system-level judgements will, for example, partly flow from ideological assumptions about how far healthcare provision should be marketized, but they will also flow from the prevailing complex of specific and deliberate health strategies. Institutional regimes will partly be an attempt to realize the value set of the system but will, necessarily, refract and add to this value set. This is why I said at the beginning of the Preface that we can only make appraisals of professional ethics in the light of 'institutional ethics' and 'policy ethics'. Generally I am arguing that ethical analyses need to work at these three levels and take into account the inter-actions between them. What, for example, are the ethical implications for health services and for clinical encounters if we adopt a system commitment to the reduction of health inequalities?

But what can I mean by appraisal here? An ethical analysis cannot simply *describe* interactions between levels. Once we go down the road of talking about social construction or value fields, do we not leave the task of ethics behind? Looking at social contexts may be of some interest but it is not doing the traditional job of applied ethics—that is deciding upon the defensibility of ethical claims. Furthermore once we acknowledge that value judgements are a product of social and cultural systems does not some kind of relativism automatically follow? We may be left with the ability to appreciate why certain judgements have been made in a particular context but we cannot judge those judgements. In the hope of achieving some kind of greater sensitivity we will have given up the game completely. We will be left with rival cultures and enhanced cultural understanding but without the inde-pendent reasoning tools to evaluate or make recommendations.

Hence the importance of the questions raised above about the role of healthcare ethics 'reason' in relation to practical rationality within specific systems and contexts. This concern that a focus on 'cultures' undermines the proper focus on independent reasoning and questioning in healthcare ethics is, it seems to me, the principal objection that many applied philosophers have to the increasing prominence given to the social sciences, and to empir-ical work specifically, within healthcare ethics. Much of this attention to social science questions is—it is thought—simply beside the point. What matters is not descriptions but evaluations; not accounts of how things are but of how they *ought* to be, and the latter requires an independent delibera-tive healthcare ethics that is rooted in moral philosophical debate, and no amount of empirical work can substitute for this. Against this how would I defend my emphasis upon the importance of social reflexivity? In large measure I would want to defend the importance of a socially reflexive healthcare ethics through looking at how it might work in practice, and I hope some of what follows will fulfil this role. But I will say a little here by way of a general defence.

Whilst I entirely agree that it is important to keep a strong sense of whether, at any one time, we are asking descriptive or evaluative questions, I would equally want to stress the many ways in which these different kinds of question have relevance for one another. First, unless we devote time to exploring and uncovering the construction of the value field of healthcare and the competing discourses and value sets that run through it there is a danger that the critical and evaluative questions we ask will be too circumscribed; that we will—to put it baldly—take too much at face value. Second, healthcare ethics must pay some regard to the social construction of ethical ideals, obligations, and dispositions. That is to say we cannot afford only to ask in the abstract, 'what ought to be done?'; there are also important questions about the ways in which agents and 'agencies' ethical frameworks, and scope for action, are defined. This may seem to place too much weight upon what might be called 'conventional ethics', i.e. it doesn't follow from the fact that a particular health professional is not currently allowed 'to do x' or 'make y judgement' that it would not be right for them to do these things. But this objection misses the point. The point is that factors like the way roles and perspectives are defined are *relevant* to our ethical deliberations. It is relevant to making ethical judgements about *this* health professional *here and now* that they are not permitted to do these things, and should we propose that the frameworks which define their role should change then these new frameworks would be relevant to appraising their actions. Third, this example indicates a more general phenomenon, namely that questions about 'what is possible' are central to ethical appraisal but are questions which depend upon the kinds of descriptive and explanatory work that can only be approached through social scientific and empirical work. There is very little to be gained by asserting that we can reconcile the apparent tension between value A and value B *in principle*, if we have absolutely no idea how we might go about doing so in practice, or even whether or not it is possible to do so. Fourth and finally, and I won't be pursuing this more philosophical line of thought in this book, there may well be, therefore, much deeper epistemological and methodological linkages between ethical and empirical questions. It may be that ethical theory, if it is to be defensible, can only be framed against some empirically informed understanding of the possibilities and limits of social action and social change.

In outline my view is that the deliberative ethics fostered by analytic applied ethics—an approach to ethics which takes seriously the task of discriminating between and defending substantive ethical claims—needs to incorporate a sociologically informed 'critical ethics'. By 'critical ethics'

I mean an approach to the value field of health policy and healthcare which not only describes the values represented (whenever necessary drawing upon empirical work to do so) but also moves towards evaluations of the intended and unintended effects of these values. Just as descriptive ethics without a harder evaluative edge tends towards relativism, a deliberative ethics which lacks a critical consciousness about the social context of health will tend towards abstract rationalism. This means, amongst other things that it will tend to work *within* rather than work *on* the constitution of whatever happens to be the prevailing value field.

I will try to illustrate this combination of deliberative and critical perspectives in the following two chapters in which I reflect more closely on what are arguably the two core substantive issues raised by the diffusion of the health agenda. First, what are the ends of health policy and second, how far can the locus of health-related decision-making move away from 'the experts' or the relevant authority figures? In both cases these questions connect with important discursive shifts in health policy, discourses around holism or positive health, for instance, or around partnership and empowerment. What are some of the values represented by these discursive shifts, and how ought we to evaluate them and their effects?

2

Producing the Goods: Health, Welfare and Well-being

How can we produce the goods when it comes to health? Prominent discourses around economic efficiency and evidence-based healthcare, along with the technicism that often lies behind them, point up the importance of maximizing 'health outcomes'. But what I have called the diffusion of the health agenda—the emphases both on broader determinants and also on culture and subjectivity as well as biology—creates problems about the boundaries and ends of health systems. Once we move beyond a narrow biomedical model we become less certain about what counts as, and what produces, 'health goods', and less certain about what counts as health work and what health work is for. In this chapter I want to explore some of these uncertainties. One way of approaching these concerns is through the concept of health and this is the focus of the first half of the chapter. But, as will become clear as I proceed, this sort of 'definitional' work is insufficient on its own. It is also important to consider the ways in which various conceptions of health or other health-related goods are, or ought to be, embodied in policies and practices, as self-consciously chosen ends or as elements built into the value field. (Because what matters, ultimately, is not what we take health-related concepts to mean but what kinds of, and distribution of, goods are produced by the social processes in which these concepts are embedded.) In the second part of the chapter I want to ask some more direct questions about the nature and boundaries of healthcare and health policy, about the difficulties of isolating health from health-related goods, or health-related goods from other goods, and about some of the value tensions inherent in health-related discourses

Health professionals tend not to think much about 'health'. This is for a very good reason. They are normally too busy doing specific things with specific ends in sight, for example, reassuring someone, making them more comfortable, vaccinating them, excising a tumour, prescribing pain killers, or giving dietary advice. There are obviously countless healthcare activities such as these, which can be combined in packages and trajectories of care, or which can be further broken down into component practices which rest upon specific sets of skills and knowledge. There is an important sense in which thinking about health in the midst of this is 'beside the point'. Healthcare is merely a loose organizing category which bundles these diverse practices together, and health is merely a useful compound label for what they are all directed towards.

If we start from health policy, however, things are somewhat different. Particularly given the diffusion of the health agenda, and the accompanying social reflexivity, health policy-makers are necessarily conscious of 'health' as an end. Policy-making places more emphasis on the word 'health', and at least some of the time it does so with the implication that health is not necessarily the same thing as whatever 'healthcare' happens to aim at. Some people involved with the health-promotion movement, for example, see the movement as reflecting a critique of the goals of traditional healthcare precisely because these centre around disease management rather than the creation of health. Of course health policy cannot be confined to the pursuit of a single end (called 'health' or anything else)—the support, organization and regulation of healthcare and health professionals are obviously major functions of health policy, and as I have just noted these things serve a complex of ends.

How can we best understand health-related goods? Is there much to be gained by focusing our attention on the nature of health itself? If we understood more about health would we be in a better position to plan and evaluate health systems or frame public policy in general? By the end of this chapter I will have given fuller answers to these questions but I can say immediately that my response to them is a qualified 'yes'. I think the search for 'health' is a worthwhile one for health policy but is one which has limited benefits for constructing policy. In brief my reasons for scepticism are: (i) that I doubt we could approach agreement about a sufficiently circumscribed conception of health to inform health policy; (ii) that in any case health policy and healthcare are about more than the promotion of health; and (iii) that 'health-related goods' and other goods are so mutually implicated that the former cannot be dealt with in isolation. I will expand on these points as I continue. However, I suggest that reflecting on conceptions of health and health-related goods is of practical benefit because it enables us to review the ends of health policy and to critically interrogate the assumptions about ends embedded in policies and practices.

Rather than debate the meaning of health at length I will set out three ideal types of health: health as absence of disease, health as welfare, and health as well-being. These are not presented here as a serious attempt to define health but largely as a means of opening up the relevant issues. Each of them contains unresolved ambiguities and conflicts, and the terms I use for them are adopted purely for the purposes of presentation. However, they each serve to summarize and indicate a cluster of related conceptions[1]. Other people would no doubt put conceptions together into different clusters but I hope my choice is both intelligible and plausible.

Health as the absence of disease. This is the dominant biomedical conception of health. It is clearly hugely influential in all health-related debates and policy. Healthcare is often equated with disease management and there is no doubt that diseases represent harms and that alleviating their effects is a valuable activity. According to some of the advocates of this conception it offers a scientific and largely value-neutral means of determining the state of an individual's or population's health. The best-known example is Boorse's biostatistical concept of disease (1977) which defines pathology purely in relation to the biological sciences. Although Boorse's account is controversial his broad project is of first-rate importance. At least in modern Western health polities many people work with the presupposition that medical science can potentially provide an authoritative and definitive account of health and disease. This background presupposition often applies to patients as well as doctors. Something like the following thought might go through the mind of a patient visiting a doctor, 'I know I don't *feel* well but is there anything *actually wrong* with me?' Here the patient has as much of an interest in scientific objectivity as the doctor. The belief that the tools of medical science can 'cut through' the uncertainties of our private experiences, in principle if not always in practice, itself provides one of the functions of biomedicine, i.e. helping to offer definitive insight into our biological constitution.

But the convergence of the medical science and lay agendas has limits. The thinking summarized above, which contrasts the patient's 'feelings' with the doctor's 'objective' diagnosis, makes this clear. In many respects the categories of medicine are alien to the experiences of health and disease. They may purport to explain our experiences but they do not 'capture' them. Sociologists summarize this distinction between the scientific and the phenomenological perspectives in the distinction between disease and illness. Illness is what we suffer from (whether or not caused by an identifiable biological dysfunction) and illness transcends the categories of medicine in a number of respects. Our illness or 'dis-ease' includes not only 'bad sensations', aches and pains, and so on, but also the experience and continued threat of 'biographical disruption' (Radley, 1983; Williams, 1989). When we are ill we cannot do all the things we wish to do, our plans are held in check or are subject to revision. With serious acute or chronic illness our whole life-plans,

---

[1] I have worked with these constructions before (Cribb, 2002) but the formulation and discussion of them in this chapter is also informed by conversations with George Khushf about his work on concepts of health (Khushf and McKeown, 2000, and Khushf, 2001).

identities, and relationships are threatened in a sometimes turbulent sea of fear and hope. A healthcare system, or a doctor, that ignored these aspects of illness would be a very poor one indeed. And, as I noted in Chapter 1, the biomedical model is increasingly qualified in practice by a response to individual subjectivity and agency.

Thus a healthcare system framed around this first conception of health would concentrate upon all aspects of disease management (prevention, cure, symptom control). In practice this will inevitably include some systems for managing the 'phenomenological correlates' of disease. However, once we allow illness and not simply disease into the picture we also have to reconcile qualitatively different perspectives and priorities. Medical *practice* must be sensitive to individual and culturally specific constructs of health, and some health professionals will take seriously the need for 'narrative reconstruction' following illness, but medical *science* does not pretend to encompass these things. There is a danger that the objectivity and determinacy of biomedicine will unravel if 'health' concerns are defined too broadly. By contrast if we define health as the absence of disease it may be possible to provide a solid anchor point to delimit the proper concerns of medical science and the core rationale of medical practice.

Health as welfare. As we have seen defining health as the absence of disease allows us to develop a relatively objective and value-neutral conception but it creates other problems. It provides a very thin conception of health which not only fails to reflect the many thicker conceptions in everyday use but even fails to represent that subset of conceptions common in healthcare practice. Here to be restored to health is to 'feel better' and to be able to resume 'normal activities', to have the phenomenological and biographical disruptions of illness repaired or 'healed'. None of these ideas can be properly captured in the language of disease. This suggests the need for a broader, and perhaps a more positively conceived, conception of health where health is defined in terms of the ability to live one's life.

I have labelled this broader idea of health 'welfare' and am deliberately trading on the associations between 'welfare' and 'welfare policies' or the 'welfare state'. In these uses 'welfare' picks out something like a necessary minimum of well-being. To provide welfare is to provide a platform of goods and services which enables individuals to live their own lives and participate in society. To lack welfare is to be 'needy', to have welfare is to have one's basic needs met, to have the resources to achieve greater well-being. Some accounts of health certainly overlap with this notion of welfare. Parsons defined the health of an individual as the capacity to fulfil the 'role and tasks for which he has been socialized' (1981: 69) and WHO have described health as 'a resource for everyday living' (1986). These accounts, and similar ones which equate health with an ability, or capacity, or set of resources present a more positive conception of health, and one which connects it to the life-world and social world and not only the biological world. As I have indicated this picture reflects many common-sense uses but it has also been elucidated in various philosophical accounts of health. For example those of Seedhouse (2001) and Nordenfelt (1987).

Seedhouse describes health as follows, 'A person's optimum state of health is equivalent to the state of the set of conditions which fulfil or enable a person to work to fulfil his or her realistic chosen and biological potentials' (2001: 84). Nordenfelt describes health as 'the ability to realize vital goals', where vital goals are defined as those necessary to achieve minimal happiness. I cannot do justice to these different accounts, or the arguments lying behind them, but I would like to make a few points about them which relate to the immediate task of mapping conceptions of health. These welfare versions of health make it dependent upon broader ideas like fulfilment, happiness, or well-being. Unless we can give some general account of what I am calling 'well-being' we cannot identify whether or not the conditions necessary for well-being are in place. This decisively moves the discussion of health away from the relatively value-neutral domain of biological science and into the heart of evaluation. In brief the presence of health is indicated by the presence of, or potential for, a valuable life. How then can advocates of a welfare conception prevent the idea of health being swallowed up in highly contested conceptions of well-being, or getting bogged down in endless debates about the nature of a worthwhile or happy life?

Both Seedhouse and Nordenfelt use the same two basic moves here (albeit within two different frameworks). First, they stress the minimal scope of their focus when talking about health—they are, roughly speaking, only referring to the conditions for autonomy. Precisely what is needed to establish autonomy may in practice vary from person to person but we can employ general criteria for autonomy which need not embody thick conceptions of well-being. Second, they explicitly rule out the 'external imposition' of thick conceptions of well-being by stipulating that any determination of 'fulfilled potentials' or 'minimal happiness' is made in relation to the choices and preferences of the individual concerned. I will not discuss the success or failure of these moves here but I will come back to these sorts of manoeuvres because they represent a key issue in health policy—the possibility of separating off the 'foundations' for social life, or what are sometimes called 'primary goods' (Rawls, 1972: 92–3) from the debates about what makes life worth living.

The welfare conception of health may capture some of our ordinary intuitions in making health more than the absence of disease but, perhaps because the biomedical model is integrated into lay perspectives, it may seem to jar with others. Does not identifying health with the conditions for autonomy not make it too broad? Are there not all kinds of things which provide a platform for action which seem to fall outside the scope of health? For example, a certain measure of wealth or income, a certain level of education, perhaps a certain compound of opportunities are all arguably necessary for achieving well-being (or even for achieving thresholds for autonomy on some interpretations). These may all be encompassed by the idea of welfare as it is used in expressions like 'the welfare state', they all meet basic needs and are therefore important goods for public policy to consider. But that does not make them 'health'. Of course they may all also be *determinants* of health, but we must be careful to distinguish between the determinants of health and health itself. There is an ambiguity here between health as welfare and health as a component of welfare. It is worth noting that Seedhouse's and Nordenfelt's accounts diverge at this point. Seedhouse equates health with what I have called welfare and Nordenfelt equates it only with a component of welfare. Seedhouse wishes to replace the focus on disease with a focus on welfare in general and he is quite prepared to 'stretch' the meaning of health in the process. Nordenfelt does not consider external resources to play a constitutive role in his conception of health. He restricts his account to the internal or 'constitutional' resources of the individual. In so doing he builds a bridge between the broader welfare conception and the disease-oriented conceptions of health, but with the former playing the primary role. Welfare provides the rationale which allows us to determine what counts as pathology.

Health as well-being. The most well-known definition of health is that used in the Constitution of the World Health Organization (WHO, 1946): 'Health is a state of complete well-being, physical, social and mental, and not merely the absence of disease or infirmity.' This definition has some of the same advantages as those rehearsed under the welfare conception. It captures the positive connotations of health in everyday discourse, and in particular it suggests that there are ideals of health and not merely degrees of freedom from disease. Of course it has also been the object of much criticism for its unqualified idealism and vagueness. The central criticism can be put in the form of a question: 'How could we use this definition to judge the standard of health of an individual or a population?' Even assuming that this definition allows for degrees of health short of 'complete well-being' we have very little to go on. There are so many ambiguities. For example is well-being something that I just 'enjoy' when, perhaps I am full of life and feel things are going well, or do certain conditions—which?—have to be satisfied? Are any such conditions 'personal' or 'impersonal': do I have well-being if I meet my own criteria, or do I have to meet some external 'objective' standard? But the fact that this famous definition raises problems of interpretation is not a reason to dismiss the conception of health as well-being. It simply indicates that if we want to take this conception seriously there is much more work to be done.

And there may be reasons, apart from its endorsement by WHO, to take this conception of health seriously. At the level of public policy a concern with health is not always clearly separated off from broader concerns with well-being. Welfare and other public policies that seek to build infrastructures, improve environments or tackle social exclusion, for example, are directed at a wide variety of goods which include health. And these separations cannot be made easily even within healthcare. Health professionals often do use some quite general terms when describing the scope and purpose of their work. They talk, for example, about the patient's (or group's) interests, benefit, or quality of life. They do not by any means restrict their attention to 'optimum disease management', rather this focus is mediated through the wider considerations indicated by these more general terms. It is in a patient's interests to have their wishes respected even if this makes their disease state worse. A patient can benefit from having access to reading matter or television even if these things have no impact on their medical condition. Quality of life may be improved by moving patients to an environment in which they feel more comfortable, or one which allows them to pursue personal projects, even if this undermines their prognoses. These are all commonplace occurrences and ones which suggest that the proper focus of healthcare is well-being. (I will return to the relationship between what I am calling welfare and well-being later but in these examples something more than welfare is in play: the television in the second example or the comfort in the third example may not amount to 'basic needs'.) If healthcare is 'about' well-being then why not simply define health as well-being? We could then concentrate on explicating the concept of well-being.

A moment's reflection shows why this definitional step will not do. Many things are 'about' well-being—education, the arts, family relationships, and so on. This does not mean that they can all be defined as well-being! Furthermore the fact that health professionals must have regard to well-being is an important one, but it is not an argument for equating health and well-being. It seems more plausible to say that health makes a contribution to well-being, but that health professionals need to take into account the effects of their actions on both health and other aspects of well-being. It is equally clear that, in practice, health-professional activity is primarily aimed at some subset of well-being-related goods: it is not, for example, aimed at aesthetic satisfaction or educational attainment. Making these distinctions between goods is vital if we are to make any evaluations of healthcare. Unless we have the conceptual resources to distinguish between different sorts of goods we cannot even frame the sorts of choices mentioned above between 'health' or wishes, 'health' or comfort, etc. There is also a place for comprehensive judgements that life is 'going well' but, again, these comprehensive judgements cannot be made if all of the possible constituents of such a life are fudged together into a single overarching but indeterminate good.

But this line of argument raises further questions. First, in order to make a distinction between health and well-being I must be relying on some notion of these two terms. In particular if health is not to be equated with well-being we need an alternative account of health, and if health professionals are also to take into account well-being we need some conception of this. Second, given that 'quality of life', in some version, is a goal for health-professional work we need to decide whether or not something like this should fall within our account of health or whether it is a supplementary good. Third, the emphasis I have placed on what health professionals happen to do or think, or on our everyday intuitions about the meaning of health, raises the question of whether these things ought to be revised. Is it not possible that we could give a defensible account of the meaning of health—perhaps quite a broad account—which would then enable us to reform healthcare practices accordingly? As I have noted this is part of Seedhouse's project and, more widely, it is a hope expressed by many advocates of health promotion.

I will assume that, for the reasons rehearsed above, health cannot be simply 'revised' to mean well-being. It is not only that this would overturn our current uses, it is also that we would lose essential discriminating power. How then are health and well-being connected? Fortunately we have in the philosophical literature some highly developed analyses of the nature of well-being which we can take as a starting point. Once again I will merely summarize some of them here (neglecting the substantial argumentative resources their authors provide).

Griffin sees well-being as 'the fulfilment of informed desires' (1986: 14), according to his analysis someone has well-being if their life satisfies what might be called their most important desires. ('Importance' here signals two aspects of Griffin's fuller account. First, the desires in question should be informed and not based on logically or empirically mistaken reasoning. Second, they contribute more to well-being to the extent that they are 'higher' in the structure of desires, i.e. are more fundamental 'desires about desires'.) Sumner defines well-being as 'authentic happiness' (1996: 172), where happiness is understood as self-evaluated life satisfaction (provided that such evaluations meet specific epistemic standards and are generally informed and autonomous). Raz defines well-being as 'the whole-hearted and successful pursuit of valuable activities' (1994: 3) and then goes on to explain and discuss each of the terms of the definition in some depth.

These three accounts are all relatively formal ones, i.e. they are consistent with a very wide range of substantive experiences of well-being. Each of these authors is aiming at an abstract and general account of what it is to have a valuable life which is compatible with qualitatively different value sets and with many different 'routes' through the combination of goods open to people. There are obviously differences between these accounts but there are also striking similarities. Each of them relates well-being to a state of affairs in which there is a 'match' between life experiences and what is (carefully) judged to be most valuable or worthwhile (at least to the person concerned). It may seem that there is something rather 'worthy' about these accounts as if only a life devoted to art or charitable works might qualify, but this is not the case. In principle the life of a narrow hedonist could qualify—it depends upon whether the judgements that underpin such an approach to life would be sustained and borne out in practice. Each of these accounts requires that subjective perceptions of value are filtered through epistemic criteria—thinking that something is valuable does not make it valuable—but each of them also allows that to some degree substantive judgements of an individual's well-being depends upon knowing something about that individual's value priorities. This sensitivity to individuality does not rule out the possibility that there are a range of well-being constituents which are shared across human beings either because their importance is 'built into' the human constitution or because they are cultural 'givens'. Raz's emphasis on the centrality of 'activity' is a possible example; and Griffin offers a longer list (including autonomy, enjoyment, loving relationships, and accomplishment) of *kinds* of good which we arguably share in common.

If, for the purposes of this discussion, we just assume that these accounts are along the right lines then what do they tell us about the relationship between health and well-being? If health is the absence of disease then it does not appear to be a significant constituent of well-being. It would seem to be a rather impoverished vision that placed 'not having a disease' as a central criterion of life's being valuable, happy, or successful. Absence of disease seems more like a condition for well-being rather than a constituent of it. Being disease-free, including being free from serious disease, is not a necessary condition of well-being. (It is quite possible to imagine 'good lives' which are accompanied by serious illness and suffering.) But, generalizing, we can say that absence of disease, especially serious, chronic, or life-threatening disease, helps to make well-being possible. And this is the idea that is made explicit in the welfare conception of health which explicitly links health to the conditions which enable the pursuit of well-being. However, as I noted above, to equate health with *all* of these conditions is to stretch its normal use enormously.

Finally, it is worth remembering that there are alternative meanings of the term 'well-being'. The above accounts are all attempts to get at a comprehensive idea of well-being, of a life going well or being worthwhile. They relate to a fundamental and long-term appraisal of life's quality. There are, of course, many more immediate ways of appraising the quality of life. My state of well-being can refer to the fact that right now, or this month, I feel good: I feel well, comfortable, joyful, and energetic. And with respect to these experiences there is no significant difference between feelings and making judgements—feeling well is all that is involved in 'judging' that I am well. In this sense many things, including healthcare, can contribute to my 'being well'. And in this sense feeling healthy does seem to be a constituent of well-being. The WHO conception of health as well-being presumably rests partly on these associations.

There is no reason to suppose that we need to fix upon a single conception of health as the right one. After all the term is used within different sets of discourses, both lay and professional, and is applied in different contexts and at different levels of abstraction, for example to both individuals and popu-lations. But it is essential to recognize the slipperiness of the concept and to have some self-consciousness about this as we use it from case to case. Hence I am not interested in settling the question of the meaning of health here but I will (in the following section) indicate how, in the main, I have chosen to interpret the term in this text.

Some people may feel that, in making these remarks about the relative open-endedness of the concept, I am being too woolly and am in danger of abandoning rigour. They may stress the need for closure, at least around some health-professional conception of health. Imagine a profession of diamond providers who said that there are simply different conceptions of what counts as a diamond and there is no authoritative account. There are, for example, lay conceptions of diamonds and sometimes, for reasons of customer service, they only provide diamonds that meet these conceptions! Here the response is obvious. Some things are diamonds and other things are not. Professional diamond providers need to be able to identify diamonds. If they provide anything else they are failing in their profession and cheating their customers. Talk of rival conceptions or contestability is hokum. Might this not be a decent analogy for healthcare? Are not health policy-makers and healthcare professionals there to 'provide' health, and is it not their business to be able to identify health unequivocally?

There is a great deal at stake here. The authority of healthcare profes-sionals depends upon their claims to expertise about health. Also systems of payment, funding, and accountability depend upon the 'purchaser' or regu-lator being provided with a certain circumscribed range of goods—who is to define, and 'assay', these goods? This is where the biomedical conception of health as disease-freedom comes strongly into play. This conception offers the possibility of an objective, essentially scientific, means of identifying levels of health and the effectiveness of services. As long as they are prepared to appoint and trust experts in medical science it gives purchasers and regulators a health measure for accountability purposes. There are thus practical and philosophical reasons to support the claim of the biomedical conception to be *the* conception of health. It seems to offer a sure foundation for health services and health policy. If we accept this foundational role for the biomedical conception of health the undoubted social power that it gives the medical profession—in defining and measuring health and all that entails—will be, at worst, a 'necessary evil'.

But there are also practical and philosophical reasons to be cautious before giving this conception free reign. First, as noted above, it is clear that health policy and healthcare, including medical practice, operates with a broader focus than disease management. Healthcare practices themselves aim at a variety of ends, including aspects of quality of life and autonomy, which are plausibly gestured towards by the label 'health' but which are not covered by the science of disease. Second, it is far from clear that diseases can be wholly defined and understood in scientific terms, especially if science is conceived as a value-neutral domain of knowledge. If diseases are conceptualized as biological abnormalities which cause deficits in functioning, then how do we decide at what level a natural variation becomes an abnormality or what counts as a deficit in functioning? It seems that the final item here—deficit in functioning—must be conceptually central and it is difficult to see how this could be anything other than a value-laden judgement. There may obviously be many cases where the value judgements involved are uncontroversial but there will be many others where this is not the case. At precisely what level does, for example, a loss of sexual functioning in an older man become pathological, or alternatively, shyness in a child, or alcohol dependency, or reduced fertility levels, or attention deficit, or shortness of height? All of these things may be partly explicable as biological deficits, and partly treatable as such, but they will no doubt have also to be defined by social judgements which will necessarily reflect historically specific cultural values.

Given that we accept, for the reasons just rehearsed, that there is a normative as well as an empirical element to disease ascriptions we are left with the issue of whether these two elements are 'inextricably intertwined' (Khushf, 2000). Might, that is, the science of diseases, be able to have a relatively autonomous existence as long as we acknowledge the role played at the margins by social valuations, or is it permeated with such valuations? The relationship between scientific judgements and wider social judgements is in part a much wider debate in philosophy of science and the sociology of knowledge which I will not pursue here. But I do, once more, wish to stress the crucial import of these sorts of debate for health policy.

Before moving on to consider the relevance of these definitional questions about health concepts to health policy and practice I want to stress, once more, that much of this relevance is indirect. That is, we should not only be thinking about the ways in which these concepts, or related concepts, are deliberately used in the shaping of policies and practices. Of at least equal importance is the question of how the elements of what I am calling health, welfare, and well-being are socially embedded in the constraints, cultures, organizational frameworks, and practices of healthcare. The values represented by health concepts are, of course, a central component of the value field of health-related action and here, as elsewhere, the construction of the value field can only partly be understood as a product of planning. What is needed, and I am only touching upon this here, is some reflection on, and unpacking of, the actual ends that are built into the value fields of healthcare policies and practices.

The Separability of Health and Health Policy

One way of highlighting the significance of the value dimension of health concepts is to ask the following (rather crude) questions: Can we make a clear distinction between health and other goods? Is health different? Is health, perhaps, 'objectively' good? If so this makes it easier to make sharp distinctions between areas of policy-making. We could, for example, plan health-promotion interventions with the expectation that their goal would be uncontroversial because health is a simple, universally recognized, and basic good. By comparison policies aimed at political literacy or homosexual equality, etc. would be matters of high controversy. Of course our policies might have 'side effects' on other goods but in so far as the policies were successful in promoting health they could be universally approved. We might also, on this basis, make distinctions about how to invest public money in different kinds of goods, and the principles by which it should be invested. We could, for example, argue for a certain measure of equity with regard to health, or at least a certain minimum of provision, which we might not do with other goods such as access to football or opera. More specifically, following this line of thought, we could see a 'health deficit' as grounds for some sort of social entitlement without necessarily extending this thought to other policy areas.

These thoughts are deliberately vague and hypothetical but they are merely meant to convey the kind of role that appeals to health can and do play in policy discourses. These kinds of thoughts lie behind many real world welfare policies. The common emphasis on efficiency and on designing healthcare interventions to maximize 'health outcomes' rests on these vague background assumptions. Moreover vagueness is not merely a contingent property of policy discourse which often works through image, 'feel', and association as well as by rational argument. In practice health-policy debates are often differentiated from other policy debates; this differentiation is underpinned by an image of health as a basic uncontroversial good and, in turn, this image is supported by its associations with the value-neutral authority of medical science. If health can, even in principle, be specified with this disinterested authority then some of these wider policy moves are given added plausibility. If not, then the structure of associations falls down.

In practice, as I argue below, I cannot see that the existence of a value-neutral and definitive ground would make a huge difference to most questions of macro-health policy beyond this important rhetorical issue. However, the existence of a 'relatively determinate' ground does seem to me to be of great importance. If we cannot specify health then how can we prevent health policy unravelling into debate about its scope and about rival conceptions of health? If we cannot agree on the subject matter we are discussing then how could we ever make any progress?

To some extent this process of unravelling has actually happened. The shift away from a definitive conception of health is implicit in what I have described as the diffusion of the health agenda. But it seems to me that this does not rule out the possibility of relative determinacy, and arguably makes it even more important. For that reason I will mainly use the word 'health' to refer to a relatively narrow range of goods. I have suggested that it cannot be equated simply with absence of disease, or welfare, or well-being because the first conception is too narrow and the other conceptions are too broad. However, it seems to me that if we stick fairly close to the biomedical conception but combine aspects of the wider conceptions with it we get close to a workable model of health which allows us to prevent some of the extremes of indeterminacy. I tend to use 'health' to refer to 'the absence of illness' where illness refers roughly to the object of healthcare practice rather than that of clinical science. Illness is clearly a contested and value-laden notion but one which is to some degree circumscribed by the interactions between biomedical and cultural judgements. Most putative bad things—poverty, ignorance, shame, injustice, jealousy, etc.—would not count as illnesses by either strict biomedical or broader cultural judgements. Yet in other instances there will be reasonable disputes both within and outside of biomedicine as to whether something should be regarded as an illness. The determinacy is only relative.

To 'define' health and illness in terms of the domain of healthcare practice is deliberately circular. The point is to make its scope subject to the continuous resolution of practical processes. It implies that there is no single vantage point from which it can be authoritatively defined. Biomedical science will inevitably play a predominant role in modern health polities. But its authority will always be subject to its explanatory power with regard to the experience and treatment of illness, and the ability of health professionals to interpret and apply it in ways which are responsive to the felt needs and preferences of lay people.

Operating with a fairly traditional and narrow conception of health allows us to distinguish health from other goods including what I have called welfare and well-being. Health can be seen as a component of welfare and, thereby, as contributing to the conditions for well-being. But confining the idea of health to this relatively determinate domain does very little to resolve the wider issues of indeterminacy and contestability in health policy because health policy must have regard to welfare and well-being as well as health. The analogy with 'diamond providers' falls down, therefore, in two respects. First, there is no autonomous 'natural science' determination of what counts as 'health' as there is for diamonds. Second, health policy and healthcare are not exclusively about 'providing health', they necessarily have broader sets of aims. To mention just a few obvious examples health policy clearly needs to take into account things like patients' wishes or public opinion, and arguably ends such as equity or solidarity, which are all different in kind to health. In this context simple notions such as 'efficiency' and 'maximizing outcomes' are automatically problematized.

These two factors mean that the kinds of rhetorical moves summarized above, which attempt to insulate health policy from supposedly more contested areas of public policy, have little substance behind them. It is not just that what counts as health is subject to value disputes, or that work 'for' health has side effects on other goods, it is also that work for health does not exist in isolation but only exists within a complex of policy or professional considerations. Health will always have to be carefully weighed against other goods. It may be a basic good but there are other goods which are equally fundamental or sometimes—like well-being—more fundamental. Policies aimed at promoting health will always have to be evaluated for their impact on the full range of goods they affect, and will always have to compete for priority with policies and programmes in other domains (which, in turn, will have health-related consequences of their own). This should be obvious but is sometimes hidden by the rhetorical stress on the primacy of health policy. Indeed it would make very little difference to these general points if a value-neutral and definitive conception of health were available. An aura of objectivity surrounding the good of health should not add any weight to judgements concerning its relative importance.

In brief, therefore, I would argue that for practical purposes it is possible to separate out the meaning of health from the wider notions of welfare and well-being, even though these goods are causally and constitutively interrelated. However, it is not possible to separate out health policy from other aspects of public policy, and especially not to give it some general, 'objective' priority. None of this is meant to imply that in many instances we cannot argue for the priority of health. It is simply that health, in general and case by case, has to compete in the 'market place' of concerns.

I can briefly illustrate this with the example of teenage pregnancy. Teenage pregnancy is often portrayed as both a social and a health 'problem'. In many ways its legitimacy as a matter of social concern is underscored by the health risks entailed (to mothers and babies). But there are clearly many other dimensions of the issue to consider including the financial costs in benefits and services, the life opportunities of young people, the sexual and reproductive freedom of teenagers, the defensibility of the age of consent, etc. If we relate the above discussion to this case I would want to say: (a) that the health arguments are to some degree contentious—it is not clear that the health risks of teenage pregnancy are higher than those of other 'at-risk' groups whose pregnancies typically have more social endorsement (e.g. older women). What counts as an acceptable level of risk appears to be a social judgement which is informed by a whole cluster of evaluations; (b) the other, also contestable, harms and benefits associated with teenage pregnancy are at least of equal importance to the health-related ones. There is no way in which the health considerations (even if they were non-contentious) could play a 'trump' role in policy debates.

The example of teenage pregnancy also shows that if we try to see health in the context of other goods and values there is a danger that we are deluged by an unmanageable web of value disputes. The biomedical and welfare conceptions of health can be seen as attempts to prevent some of this flooding. They both aim, in different ways, to specify goods which are 'uncontaminated' by value pluralism. In this chapter I have spent more time considering the biomedical conception but I would suggest that in the end neither of these conceptions can be wholly successful in this respect. They may each provide some relatively uncontentious ground and this is potentially very useful. But this relative stability is something which has so to speak to be 'earned' through the existence of agreements rather than something which can be 'fixed' by science or political philosophy. We can use the concept of health in more or less elastic ways and play up either its contestability or the measure of agreement which exists. I have chosen to stress the narrower conceptions and the existence of some closure around the convergence of biomedical and illness criteria. However, in the end, I would argue, whether we operate with a broad or narrow concept of health makes little difference to the breadth and intensity of value disputes surrounding health policy. All it does is to shift the locus of some of these disputes from outside to inside health concepts. On my preferred model many of these disputes have their centre of gravity 'outside' health concepts, but health—even understood as the absence of disease—is not insulated from evaluative struggles because it is causally and conceptually bound up with other goods.

Recognizing Health Goods

As I noted at the start of the chapter healthcare serves a broad range of goods. These can only be held together by the label 'health', at best, as a kind of shorthand. Healthcare practices have the management of illness as their principal rationale (although, of course, they also relate to other issues in biological or mental functioning) but even the management of illness encompasses many things. For example: preventive or curative interventions in disease processes; symptom control and relief; information-sharing and education; psychological support including the 'containment' of anxiety; care and companionship; and recognition and respect. If they are considered in the abstract, as they appear in this list, it seems odd to call all of the items on this list 'health goods'. Certainly many of these things have relevance outside health policy and healthcare. However, if we consider practical examples and real illness trajectories these are all goods which a person could reasonably expect to be provided, in particular respects, by a healthcare system and health professionals. They are more than simply 'ancillary concerns'. A dedicated garage mechanic might be encouraged to think about customer relations as an ancillary concern. But for most health professionals 'customer relations' are, broadly speaking, part of their core business.

Certainly this is 'speaking broadly'. We obviously have to consider specific professional roles, settings, and encounters to make judgements about which goods are central and which are peripheral. But this is precisely the point. We cannot view the healthcare system, or a particular institutional setting within it, as a machine for producing some predefined good. Before we can make judgements about what health policy, healthcare, or particular healthcare practices 'ought to be for' we need to do more than abstract analyses of the nature of health, welfare, and well-being. We need to look in concrete terms at the range of healthcare practices, the intentions and expectations that make them up, and at the goods they actually produce. This is not to suggest that healthcare practices cannot be critiqued, rather that this is the means properly to inform critique.

One aspect of this is to map the ways in which conceptions of health (as well as other goods) are embodied in healthcare interactions, institutional regimes, and wider health systems. Many of the implicit judgements which make up the value field of health-related action will be accomplished through the embedding and deployment of patterns of health concepts. This is the basis of the widespread critique of 'medical model' thinking in various contexts. More specifically we can, for example, examine the way in which specific structures and cultures favour certain goods sometimes at the expense of others. (There are, for example, accounts of life prolongation and symptom control being privileged over compassion on some 'aggressive' cancer wards.) Or we can examine the institutional embodiment and interpretation of health goods across healthcare sectors more generally. In primary healthcare, for example, there is a certain elasticity which allows doctors to work within some fairly broad dimensions of welfare and well-being whilst still being anchored in a frame set by fairly narrow health conceptions. This elasticity is needed in part because primary healthcare provides a filtering system to specialist clinical care and the filter has to be able to be open to many things even if it only allows some of them through. In many hospital settings the filtering out of many (but by no means all) welfare and well-being dimensions is even more pervasive and powerful.

Of course when it comes to practical debates about public-health policy it is necessary to be responsive to multiple conceptions of health. It is not possible to legislate for narrow approaches to be used, and individuals and communities will naturally use their own constructs of health to make their own points. It is consequently normal for these public conversations and debates to be at cross purposes. Some people will stick close to biomedical conceptions, others will use various broader conceptions. In mapping these varied conceptions Khushf (2001) has usefully elaborated this narrow–broad spectrum by showing that it can be applied across three axes. As well as (i) the 'dimensions of well-being axis that I have concentrated on (i.e. does health refer to biomedical functioning or to wider aspects of well-being?), we can look at (ii) the aetiological axis—are we talking about the biological causes of ill-health or the social, environmental, psychological, or spiritual causes as well?; (iii) the systems axis—are we referring to the health of bodily systems, individuals, families, communities, populations, the eco-system? When individuals and agencies make a reference to health they are picking out multiple points in the spaces created by these intersecting axes. We are never going to be in a position to reduce this diversity to a single univocal conception. But we do need to be able to enhance our sensitivity to this diversity, and to be self-conscious about the ways in which different health goods are conceptually constructed and institutionally embodied. And when we are arguing about health policy we should not rely on lazy references to the good of health but rather attempt to specify what kinds of goods are at stake in particular instances.

Health and the Public Good

One important question, for my purposes at least, is the extent to which the discourses, strategies, and measures of 'health' embodied or used in specific sectors and settings encompass what might be called 'social goods' as well as individual goods. This allows me to return briefly, by way of a conclusion to this chapter, to the main substantive (rather than methodological) theme of this book—health as a social good. I have chosen to interpret 'health' itself as the relative absence of illness, and this is essentially something enjoyed by individuals. It makes sense, therefore, to begin by stressing the importance of health as an individual good. Indeed, one might reasonably say, as a good that can *only* be enjoyed by individuals. This begs the question, 'In what sense, or senses, do I want to talk about health as a social good?'

What I am suggesting, in a nutshell, is that health is experienced primarily at the level of the individual but that the causes, content, and consequences of these health experiences are, in large measure, social phenomena. I say that health and illness is experienced 'primarily' at an individual level because even that boundary is not entirely sharp. For example, studies of the families of cancer patients reinforce what many people know from their own experience, namely that the suffering, heartache, and biographical disruption that are characteristic of serious chronic illness affect many family members and not only the patient. There is a sense in which whilst the disease is 'contained' in the individual the illness is not, but rather is experienced socially. The same thing is palpable at a community level where, for example, acts of violence, accidents, or natural disaster cause widespread injury or illness in a defined locale. In the case of infectious disease, such as in managing an outbreak of meningitis in a local school, the suffering and solidarity are combined with a shared sense of being 'at risk', and this points towards another dimension of the social nature of health which I will return to below. I do not want to trade upon some mystical seeming notion of illness seeping into the social ether. I am happy to stick by the idea that some individuals are ill and that others are not, however much they may be affected by, or at risk from, these illnesses. But it should be clear from what I have said in this chapter that whilst it may be possible, indeed necessary, to make analytical distinctions between health and other goods it is very difficult to separate health from other goods in practice, and these examples are merely one further illustration of this fact.

It is because health can be neither causally nor constitutively separated from well-being that we ought to think of health as a social good or, more strictly, as a set of social goods. Illness would not have the significance it does if it did not affect people's chances of living lives they value. Its importance, its seriousness, is dependent upon the extent to which it is linked to well-being, and this, in turn, is in many respects dependent upon the social context of health and illness. The determinants of our health, how we are treated when we are ill, who cares for us and, not least, how we are cared for—all of these things affect the experience of health and illness, and all of these things point away from the individual and to the social.

This provides us with at least three senses in which we can construe health as a social good. First, there is the sense in which we can combine assessments of individual health into population assessments, i.e. build aggregative and / or distributive judgements into health assessment. To the extent that we have regard to the overall levels of health in a population, or to the distribution of health experiences, we are treating health as a social good. Much of the work in public-health assessment falls into this category. In this case to talk about public health is merely to talk about the health status of many individuals, or of patterns of health status between groups of individuals. But there are also broader possibilities here which give rise to the two other, and overlapping, senses in which health can be construed as a social good. We can open up these possibilities by noting some of the relationships between health and the public good.

Public health is obviously not the same as the public good, but we can think of public health as part of the public good, and this makes a difference. Certainly there are more things to the public good than health. There are all of the components of well-being to consider at both the individual and collective level. How we interpret these depends both on our account of well-being and on our theory of the good society. But many theorists would stress the role of social frameworks in providing the opportunities for individual flourishing. Health is no exception. The physical and cultural environment can be more or less 'health supporting' in relation to both prevention and care; and these factors have necessarily to be addressed collectively (in some respects at least). This is the sense in which we talk about 'healthy environments' or 'healthy policies', where 'healthy' means 'health causing' or 'conducive to health'. This is not to suggest that the locus of responsibility for an individual's health or well-being falls entirely beyond the individual. Accounts of well-being typically stress the importance of activity, achievement, autonomy, and personal responsibility for well-being. As these things cannot, by definition, be 'taken over' by social arrangements; all that the latter can do in this regard is to provide, or at least protect, opportunities for them.

Other theorists, typically those of a communitarian disposition, highlight another sense in which there are 'social goods', i.e. not just aggregates, patterns, or conditions of the good things experienced by individuals separately, but rather goods which, so to speak, inhere in our sociality. They will, for example, point to the fundamental importance of relationship, mutuality, and collective identity to personal identity and well-being. They are likely to stress the role of social arrangements in providing forms of 'social capital' or solidarity. These are social goods, in other words, which transcend the simple aggregative or distributive model. These are public goods in the more technical sense of the term, i.e. they are goods that are by their nature indivisible—shared goods which cannot be 'shared out'. Now health as I have interpreted it is not, strictly speaking, a social good in the way that, say, clean air or public buildings are, although I hope the examples rehearsed above suggest some strong analogies with these things. However, all of those institutions, relationships, and practices which are designed to support health can be seen as social goods in this sense. They are one of the fundamental respects in which mutuality is socially embodied.

Hence if we move from the consideration of 'health status' to thinking about health experiences in social context, then all of the themes just discussed are directly relevant. In addition to asking about the overall levels or patterns of health, we can also ask about (i) the protection, provision, and distribution of 'health opportunities' and (ii) the extent to which social provision reflects or embodies forms of mutuality or solidarity. (This latter because even though health itself is not a relational good, healthcare and health policy can be seen in this way.) This gives us a variety of ways in which, even where health is understood quite narrowly, the good of health can be treated as a social good.

These remarks help to explain my choice of title for this book. I am hoping to point to public-health matters as the essential context for approaching healthcare ethics. But I would not want 'public-health matters' here to be understood narrowly (i.e. as about the management of population levels of morbidity and mortality). Rather I am thinking about the relationship between health and the public good, whilst recognizing the contestability of the notion 'public good', to signal the relevant framework for analysis in healthcare ethics. This framework, I am suggesting, opens up a package of broad ethical debates and dilemmas which lie behind all deliberations in healthcare ethics. It is not just the permanent balancing act between individual and population benefits and harms we have to think about. We also have to think about the ways in which we, individually and collectively, create fairer opportunities to experience health, and about how far the policies and practices we are implicated in embody the kinds of relationships and social identities we value. I will return to these themes in subsequent chapters but first I need to ask some questions about the 'we' in the preceding sentences. How far does it make sense to talk about 'our responsibility' here when healthcare is controlled by some and not by others?

3

Participating in Health Decisions: Patient and Community Empowerment

The diffusion of the health agenda involves rhetorical and actual shifts in all of the value fields surrounding health, including the associated 'fields of power'. The 'widening' and 'deepening' of the agenda mean that broader sets of agents and agencies are seen as health-related actors. Our increased understanding of the social determinants of ill-health, of the limitations of health services, and of the cultural and biographical construction of health-related experiences all place health-professional power in context. Indeed, one key manifestation of the evolution of power relations—a manifestation linked to wider economic, social, and organizational changes over the last fifty years—has been the reconstruction of professional power both in relation to clients or consumers on the one hand and to budget holders and managers on the other. The work of health professionals is increasingly under the control or influence of others; and these changes have been partly accomplished through discourses of participation.

At the professional-client level these change have been played out in the shift in emphasis, in short, away from professional paternalism and towards patient autonomy. Similarly in many health-policy contexts there is a regular call for community 'empowerment'. Empowerment is summoned up not merely as something desirable but as something transformational, something with the potential to improve and legitimate health-related decision-making. Obviously we should be sceptical about all such sweeping ideas. The dangers are twofold: that these are merely linguistic shifts working only as 'spin' and masking the persistence of other values and power relations, or that to the extent that the shifts are actually embedded in practice this may, in any case, be at the expense of other valuable things. The discussion in this chapter will illustrate the relevance of both of these dangers. I want to consider the impetus behind this championing of empowerment, and to look beyond its rhetorical importance to assess its substantive importance and its limitations. I am exploring these questions about participation and empowerment in order to complete my review of the diffusion of the health agenda and the associated changes to the value fields of healthcare. The focus upon health-related decisions and processes is meant to complement the focus on 'ends' in the previous chapter, but I will include some reminders that substantive and process issues are not so easily separated out.

Lying behind the immediate focus on participation in decision-making is therefore the fundamental matter of the distribution of and use of power. In modern health polities vast amounts of human energy and financial resources are deliberately directed at health through healthcare systems and health-promotion policies. The actual and potential effects of these systems and policies on individual people's lives and on the distribution of life chances and welfare are colossal. And the proper basis for control and direction of these resources is therefore undoubtedly a crucial moral and political question.

In this chapter I am using the idea of power in a very broad sense to encompass what might sometimes be better referred to as authority. In saying that the language of empowerment is often used to 'legitimate' things I am relying upon the notion that power-sharing has an ethical value and, more specifically, that this ethical value consists in part in providing a more defensible authorization of decision-making. The empowerment movement coincides with a putative shift from expert authority to more democratic forms of authority. Power refers to those forces which shape the possibilities and contours of action, either, as I noted above, through the determinations of de facto powerful social actors (rulers, bosses, parents, etc.) or through the more diffuse influence of discursive regimes. Talk of 'authority', by contrast, relies on the judgement that the influence of certain social actors or 'ways of proceeding' is legitimate. We might judge, for example, that doctors and pharmacists should have more power over the distribution of medicines than other people. Their relevant expertise, the fact that they are in this different sense authoritative, arguably supports their relative authority in this domain. But the increasing emphasis on democratic authority encourages us to qualify this judgement in two respects. First, the fact that a doctor may have some authority over the dissemination and availability of a medicine does not necessarily encompass authority over the patient with regard to the use of the medicine. There is less scope now for the slippage of authority relations from one domain to another. Second, as I discussed in the opening chapter, the fact that medical science and the professional organizations of medicine have considerable authority over medicines is not the end of the matter. There is now a widespread appreciation of the social and political construction of medical authority and of the need to regulate the use of that authority.

So who can and should decide what is done and what is not done in the name of health? Whether in relation to individual doctor–patient encounters or in health-related public policy this question has become prominent in both popular and academic discourse. The question can be presented in a number of different forms and can be related to very different value concerns and to different facets of healthcare. But, in brief, an increased role for participation in healthcare decisions has been advocated on the basis of both effectiveness and respect for persons. If a health professional or policy-maker wants to benefit me or my community then they arguably have to acquire some 'local knowledge', including knowledge of client values and preferences. (Indeed some forms of 'care' consist of these sorts of attention and responsiveness.) Equally, given certain assumptions about the importance of mutual respect and democratic values, if a health intervention is designed to affect me, directly or indirectly, then it is 'only right' that I have a chance to participate in its design.

In what follows I will review the nature and ethical significance of participation in both healthcare and health policy. In the process I will also have in mind the relationship between participation at the levels of care and policy, including the relationship between people participating as patients and as citizens. The discussion is designed not only to highlight the central ethical importance of participation, but also to specify the reasons it falls far short of an 'ethical panacea'. Participation has to be understood as only one element in a complex nexus of competing healthcare goods.

One-to-One: From Informed Consent to Shared Decision-making

There are many ways in which individual patients are 'involved' in the decisions of their doctors[1], not all of which would count as participation in any rich sense. In consultations private biological and biographical facts are accessible to the doctor, and the patient's body and mind are routinely 'handled' and laid bare. Medical records, imaging techniques, and bodily samples mean that this accessibility continues in important respects when the patient is no longer in the same room. So patients are involved in at least the same way that the subjects of newspapers articles are involved in the stories written about them: they are implicated and they are affected.

Beyond this doctors will necessarily 'take into account' facts about their patients, including facts about their beliefs, cultural perspectives, and preferences, in brief the patient's 'values'. We might say that in this way the patient's preferences 'contribute' to the decision-making process. They are of relevance and are treated as such. But, in these cases, we might say that the preferences contribute but the patient does not. There is, as yet, no sense of

---

[1] In this section I will talk about 'doctors' as a key example of 'health professionals'. I will be deliberately engaging in broad generalizations. Of course the issues surrounding participation and power will differ significantly from professional group to group, across social and institutional settings, and also from specialism to specialism within professional groups. These are just some dimensions of the social construction and embeddedness of professional roles which I will consider later in the chapter and discuss further in Part 3.

the patient being a party to the decision-making. This is not surprising because up to now the scene has been framed solely in terms of the doctor's agency with the focus upon clinical decision-making. If we consider the broader picture there is inevitably a place for the patient's agency as well.

Typically it is the patient who initiates the consultation. He or she decides to present some concerns to the doctor and often to ask certain things of the doctor. He or she chooses to respond to the doctor's questions and to accede to investigations. Following the consultation the patient normally has a choice about whether or not to 'comply' with the doctor's advice or prescriptions. Analysing participation in healthcare requires more than taking snapshots of clinical decisions. In the normal circumstance of modern healthcare it would simply be a mistake to represent the patient as a mere 'object' wholly subject to the power of the doctor. Nonetheless safeguards are demanded by the fact that in many specific circumstances the relative vulnerability of the patient and the relative power of the doctor risk this kind of professional domination.

The language and practices of informed consent are now established as the basic safeguard of patients' interests in healthcare decision-making. It is not enough for the patient's 'self' or agency to be involved in healthcare processes. It is ethically necessary for patient's to be party to clinical decisions wherever and whenever they are in a position to do so. According to this model there is a necessary minimum standard for patient participation, a threshold below which medical decision-making becomes ethically unacceptable. Presuming that patients are competent, are adequately informed about what is being proposed, and freely consent to it, doctors have cleared this ethical hurdle.

Accepting that certain levels of patient participation are ethically necessary are greater levels not ethically desirable? This certainly seems to be the thrust of movements such as 'patient-centred' or 'person-centred' healthcare. Person-centredness is often left undefined and could itself be subject to extended analysis but I will confine myself to distinguishing three possible components: (a) person-centredness as a recognition of 'individuality' or specificity; (b) person-centredness as a recognition of 'holism', i.e. of the range of considerations and contexts which are constitutive of persons; and (c) person-centredness as a recognition of autonomy, i.e. a concern to respect people as to some degree self-defining and self-creating and to work 'with' them and not just 'on' them. It would be surprising if anyone declared himself or herself opposed to person-centredness given these different possible components and the range of combinations and interpretations available. But we can imagine a rough line from the most minimal (and barely person-centred) point of paying regard to the specific biomedical complex of each individual to increasingly 'radical' interpretations which play up various dimensions of, and responses, to the second and third components. I would reserve the label person-centred for those approaches to healthcare which are some way down this line and according to which health professionals seek to respond to patients' particular personal and social circumstances and considered preferences.

The very idea of person-centredness, however, is, paradoxically, professionally centred. It is a model, which reminds the professional to be sensitive to and responsive to the client. The professional is assumed to be 'in the driving seat' and to be making decisions on behalf of the patient but in so doing they are reminded of the need to facilitate the patient's participation in the process. Models of shared decision-making have been developed to further check the influence of this professional-centredness. For example the model set out by Charles *et al.* (1997) conceives of shared decision-making as having four key elements:

1. Both the patient and the doctor are involved in the decision-making process.

2. Both parties share information.

3. Both parties take steps to build a consensus about the preferred treatment.

4. An agreement is reached on the treatment to implement.

This emphasis on consensus building and agreement is also captured in the notion of the Royal Pharmaceutical Society of Great Britain (1997) that the doctor–patient relationship should move from one based upon compliance to one based upon 'concordance'.

We see, therefore, in the move from paternalistic professionalism via informed consent to the model of shared decision-making an increasing emphasis on patient autonomy and control. The patient as a person is increasingly brought into the picture and eventually takes on the role of an equal. Doctors and patients become partners in the shared process of healthcare. The move from 'object' to 'subject' to 'equal' corresponds with the idea of patient empowerment. At least with regard to the specifics of treatment decision-making the power of the doctor is shared with the patient.

Clearly all of this is, however, a series of idealizations. Practice, which I will return to in a moment, is rather different. But these idealizations do reflect some fundamental facts about, and shifts in, the value field of healthcare. It is now widely accepted that doctors ought to treat their patients with respect and to respect their autonomous choices. This may be justified 'directly' as the recognition, demanded by any ethical system, of the equal intrinsic worth of all persons; or 'indirectly' as necessary for the promotion of certain goods such as patient welfare. Whether we place emphasis upon the intrinsic or instrumental justification for respecting patients there are certainly important instrumental benefits at stake. Patients are more likely to feel valued and cared for if they are listened to and taken notice of; the quality of decision-making is likely to be higher if it draws upon the personal knowledge and concerns of the patient; and respect for patients is, in general, more likely to engender a climate of trust and to build more effective relationships between patients and doctors. It is also possible that moves towards greater decision-making equality could help to break down some of the social distance which, in many instances, still exists between doctors and patients, which means that often vulnerable patients feel anxious, inhibited, and intimidated in their dealings with doctors.

Having acknowledged the value of patient empowerment and its potential benefits I want to move on to some more sceptical notes. These notes relate to both what is practicable and what is desirable, and to the links between these two things. (As I noted in Chapter 1 a genuinely applied healthcare ethics has to involve some consideration of what combinations of goods are 'possible', i.e. socially realizable.)

The first point to make is that the idealized model of shared decision-making about treatment described above necessarily misses out most of the real picture. This can be highlighted both by comparing it with the idea of shared decision-making in a marriage or equivalent relationship, and also by considering the ways in which all would-be partnerships are socially constructed. In a marriage-style partnership the agenda is potentially open, any and all kinds of decisions might be shared. Indeed much of the negotiation is likely to involve making decisions about decisions: what sort of decisions should the couple discuss and deliberate about? Which of the two individual's lives should be in the spotlight from moment to moment? In addition to a relatively open agenda the couple may have relatively open roles; they are not necessarily there to serve any particular functions or duties. They are not being paid to fulfil a job description or employed by a particular institution. In short the shared decision-making context is, at least in principle, a relatively free one. Of course, when we turn to real social settings, marriages may be shaped by all kinds of religious or social norms and structured, for example, by patriarchal assumptions, but here at least the liberal individualist conception of an open, free partnership of equals is, these days, at least an intelligible one. No such equivalent conception is meaningful in doctor–patient relationships.

Doctors and patients are not abstract individuals coming together to explore, define, and pursue reciprocal benefits and purposes. Any shared decision-making will be highly circumscribed by predefined agendas and by social roles and settings. To be a doctor entails filling social, professional, legal, and institutional roles. To work as a doctor entails, more or less, operating according to the structures, cultures, and priorities of medical institutions. These institutional regimes are not merely a product of the social regulation of medicine but a requirement of the even more fundamental need to establish, coordinate, and enact socially meaningful roles and relationships, in short healthcare relationships require institutional embodiment. Equally the roles and relationships of patients are in large measure defined and circumscribed by the institutional regimes of healthcare. We only have to observe a patient negotiating his/her way through a hospital, dealing with reception staff, administrators, nurses, and finally being 'allowed' to engage with doctors to be reminded of this. All of this is indeed obvious after a moment's thought, but it is so deeply embedded in our social life that it can also become invisible.

None of this is meant to imply that doctors cannot treat patients with respect, nor to suggest that there is no scope for some shared decision-making in such encounters. But focusing on the real contexts of doctor–patient interactions does raise doubts about both the practicability and, in some respects, the value of patient empowerment. The dynamics of these inter-actions are quite hard to change. The social hierarchy and social distance between many doctors and patients should not be underestimated. Also in most health systems there is a limited amount of time for consultation; and the time, through the pace and direction of the encounter, is largely managed by the doctor. If we are considering clinical decision-making, which is the focus I have chosen here, the 'point' of the consultation is, in large measure, for doctors to draw upon their expertise to offer some intervention (reassurance, information, advice, medicines, referral). This is what structures the encounter. Other agendas are, broadly speaking, 'off the point'.

Here the locus of shared decision-making is thus relatively narrow. It is the domain of what might be called health-related 'patient change' (including work done 'on' patients, patients taking medicines, patients changing their lives or minds). Given the set of possible patient changes that the doctor would recommend or endorse, there is the potential for patients to negotiate a subset which suits their understanding and preferences. This is certainly valuable and is a move on from informed consent, because patients might well be prepared to give informed consent to an alternative subset which is clinically equivalent but suits them less well. The doctor and patient can learn from one another and as a result can come to a different and better conclusion. But the involvement of the patient in clinical decision-making remains essentially a 'veto' power. The doctor's flexibility cannot extend much beyond this. The construction of their professional role means that they are not in a position to routinely allow patients to choose options outside of their recommended set, nor can they remain entirely open-minded about patients picking and choosing at will from within this set. In other words within the institutional regimes of medicine patients do not have any clear-cut entitlement to demand treatments, nor can doctors be indifferent to patients refusing treatments.

This brings to a head the limits of patient empowerment. In the arena of clinical decision-making, at least, the medical profession is not there to do what patients want, nor is it their role merely to come to an accommodation with patients' considered preferences. Doctors' functions are socially determined and, at least according to professional ideology, they are there to use their expertise to best serve patients' interests within certain constraints, and what is more they are held accountable for so doing. Of course in many cases there will be a coincidence between accommodating patients' considered preferences and serving patients' best interests. As ever the crux of the matter is only evident when they do not coincide. And the crux of the matter is that doctors, by definition, have different forms of expertise and different systems of accountabilities than patients. If they actively collude with patients in courses of action, which they have good reason to believe will be harmful to the patient (or harmful in other respects) they will be liable to blame. In particular their accountabilities extend beyond those to the immediate patient—to other affected parties, to other patients, to their employers, and to their host institutions. This is the central constraint in attempts to shift the authority of clinical judgement away from doctors and towards patients.

Doctors are forced to balance the considered preferences of patients with their reading of the patient's best interests and with these other broader constraints and considerations. To put it crudely if a patient wants to be prescribed an expensive medicine then shared decision-making may simply amount to the doctor explaining why they cannot have it! But this should not be seen as simply a resource management issue. In a fee-for-service system the doctor has to exercise exactly the same function of determining the weight that should be attached to patient preferences in the light of other goods. The doctor's role also encompasses a power of veto but it extends beyond this because doctors are legally obliged to exercise their judgement (and, for example, recommend courses of action) in a way that patients are not.

Before I conclude this section and move on to broader questions of community participation in health policy, I want to consider two critical responses to my remarks, both of which I think merit attention. First, it might be argued, my sceptical notes rely upon certain essentialist assumptions about the nature of social roles, the socio-legal status of doctors, and the institutions of medicine. In highlighting the construction of professional roles as a limit to patient empowerment should I not also pay more attention to the myriad ways in which these constructions can change and have been changing? Are not the possibilities of patient empowerment very different now than they were only twenty years ago, and should we not now be imagining new and more equal forms of partnership between doctors and patients? All of this is, I believe, true but I would suggest it is not clear what it adds up to.

There is no doubt that things are changing. The general social climate has shifted against deference to authority in every sphere. Patients are quite properly aware of their rights to information and choice. Indeed, patient organizations, the media, and new Information Technologies put them in a much stronger position to make informed demands. The social distances between doctors and patients are, in many cases, narrower. Many groups of patients are knowledgeable and confident. Some groups, such as HIV/ AIDS patients in certain settings, are also politically organized and represented in ways which make working partnerships with health-professional groups realistic. The composition of the medical profession is changing to include a broader social mix and, in particular, many more women. Doctors are subject to ever more effective 'watchdogs', which make the slide into secrecy, paternalism, or plain arrogance more difficult. Finally, there is a much more widespread recognition that good healthcare demands substantial patient involvement. All of this adds up to a social milieu in which pressing for continuing patient participation and empowerment makes sense. On the other hand the increasing regulation of medicine, accompanied by the growth of new forms of health-service management including stewardship concerns, also means that in many respects the professional and legal powers and responsibilities of doctors are ever more tightly defined. Changes to the institutional regimes of medicine which check some of the power of doctors over patients also open up new forms of administrative control over the definition and direction of doctors' work.

I will return to this issue of managerialism in healthcare in later chapters, but here I will just observe that even if changing times mean that patients have more freedom to engage with doctors it does not follow that doctors have any more freedom to engage with patients. The reverse is arguably the case. But the underlying point is that changing social circumstances may recast doctor–patient relationships in many respects but, whatever the circumstances, the possibilities of doctor–patient relationships will be socially defined and relatively determinate. They cannot be whatever we want them to be. They have to be inscribed in real social processes and institutions. In an alternative universe 'doctors' and 'patients' could have fundamentally different roles and relationships. But then these are not the doctors and patients we are currently talking about. We are talking about the doctors and patients that exist, or those that might be brought into being by currently conceivable and practicable changes. What has to be remembered is that the social construction of professional roles does not simply relate to what might be seen (by some) as 'surface' features of healthcare relationships and ethics, or features which may be more susceptible to change, e.g. classed and gendered styles of interactions and forms of social distance. It also encompasses the social realization, and institutional embodiment, of different positions in 'ethical space', in this case the different roles and responsibilities of health professionals and patients. These things are not necessarily affected by changes in styles of interaction.

The second critical response to my notes of caution about patient empowerment is about the weight I have placed upon the instrumentality of doctor–patient encounters. By focusing upon the ideal of shared decision-making, and stressing the future-oriented function of consultation around clinical decision-making and potential patient change I have failed to pay due attention to the intrinsic value of the 'meetings' of professionals and clients, and to the intrinsic value of patients being respected and properly engaged within these meetings. It would, I agree, be wrong to neglect these things. Healthcare is about respect and care as well as the production of 'health outputs'. The modern emphasis on developing doctors' communication and listening skills, in particular the importance of taking the patient's life-worlds and illness interpretations seriously is of huge intrinsic as well as instrumental importance. Furthermore if these skills are actually used they arguably shift the use of the 'consultation resource' in a direction which is more responsive to patient influence. However, I would suggest, these things do not, at least on their own, fundamentally alter the balance of power with regard to the control of clinical practice. Patients, qua patients, have a tightly circumscribed influence over clinical practice. Here there is comparatively little equality between doctors and patients and it can be argued this is not simply because greater equality in this regard is not practicable but also because it is not ethically defensible. Because, in brief, patients lack the requisite expertise and accountability to justify substantial transfers of authority. At the very least the value of greater patient involvement in healthcare decision-making has to be set against other values which might serve to qualify the emphasis it deserves.

One way of summarizing this section is to say that doctors have grounds for their decisions other than those which stem from patient involvement. These 'independent grounds' could be seen simply as the pressures and norms deriving from the institutional regimes of medicine. However, to the extent that at least some of these independent grounds and norms (e.g. those which relate to medical expertise and those which relate to the public interest) provide good reasons for clinical decision-making then they also provide some reason for limiting the transfer of authority to patients.

Many-to-Many: Consumerism, Community involvement, and Democracy

When it comes to health policy the possibilities of, and opportunities for, different sorts of participation are too complex even to mention. Following the discussions in Chapters 1 and 2 it is clear that all kinds of international, national, and local policies have potential impacts on the determinants and the experience of health; and the causal and constitutive interactions between what I have labelled health, welfare, and well-being mean that decision-making related to any aspects of human society can potentially be read as health-related decision-making. Given this, the scope for, and arguments for and against, participation in any part of public life could arguably be discussed in this section of the chapter. I will return to some of these broader themes later in the book, but here I will confine myself—simply for practical purposes—to examples of community involvement that are commonly discussed under the rubric of health policy. In brief these seem to relate to: (a) the provision and organization of clinical-health services, (b) public-health services and health promotion and, as a particular subset of these two, (c) medical and health-related social interventions which give rise to widespread public disquiet or alarm (e.g. genetic engineering, maternal surrogacy). Of course the fact that these things are the visible face of public-health policy should not be taken as a measure of their significance. There is, for example, comparatively little public discussion (compared say to discussion within sociology) of the agenda-setting power of biomedicine. It is sometimes the very fact that a discussion is less visible in the public domain that marks its significance.

Clearly the most far-reaching health-service decisions are not made within one-to-one encounters. The policy decisions which frame the health-service agenda and the settings of clinical care are made in the public domain and subject to multiple influences and agencies. In my remarks thus far, for example, I have failed to say much about patients either as consumers or as citizens. By talking about patients qua patients I have been playing up the idea of individual patients in their short-term clinical encounters with health professionals but it is also possible to use the idea of patients to refer to populations and subpopulations who have individual and collective ongoing relationships with health services in health as well as sickness.

Because my main concern is with the opportunities for increased democratic authority in healthcare decision-making I will concentrate more on patients as citizens than patients as consumers, but the force of consumerism is simply too important to ignore completely. As I have mentioned changing times mean that patients are much better placed to make effective demands on services. In addition both the existence of healthcare markets in some health polities and the installation of 'quasi-markets' (Le Grand and Bartlett, 1993) within many publicly funded services mean that patients are increasingly positioned as consumers both by health services and staff. Doctors and health-service managers need to 'keep the customer satisfied' and to attach some priority to satisfaction measures, published performance indicators, complaints, and bad press. It is perhaps in this area that there has been the most dramatic change in the fields of power which structure healthcare provision. To the extent that the doctor–patient relation is reconfigured into a provider–consumer relation then patterns of power are also reconfigured, in some respects towards the patient/consumer. Although I am not going to examine consumerism in what follows I should at least explain the reasons behind saying 'in some respects' here. It is impossible to deny that if health systems become more responsive to 'demand' then to some degree the locus of influence over decision-making shifts from providers to consumers—this is what is meant by responsiveness. However, as has often been pointed out, there are features of healthcare which should make us sceptical about blanket claims that consumerism empowers patients. Because the provision of health-care goods depends upon much specialist knowledge (at various levels, in-cluding the epidemiological and the clinical) there are significant disparities in informed decision-making capacity both globally between providers and consumers and across bodies of consumers. In relation to healthcare there is certainly the potential for individuals to concentrate their attention and pressure on demands which may not properly reflect what would be their own considered, informed, conceptions of what would be in their best inter-ests. Obviously this should not warrant unqualified paternalism but it should warrant some caution. Furthermore the always present inequalities in rele-vant knowledge and in interpersonal and socio-political influence is com-pounded in healthcare by sometimes severe inequalities in functioning due to ill-health and other vulnerabilities. This means that whilst a demand-based health economy might benefit many people it can equally leave many others with less effective power than they might otherwise have.

I would suggest that the arguments about the merits of social participation are, in many respects, analogous to the arguments rehearsed in the previous section. For example, following the discussion of one-to-one relationships above I would want to distinguish, somewhat artificially, between two faces of involvement. The passive face in which patients' concerns and preferences are 'taken into account' by health services, and the active face in which groups of patients articulate positions and make claims upon health services, in which they seek to be party to health-service decisions. For the purposes of this discussion I will assimilate the latter to the idea of patients as citizens. The passive face could be played down here because it does not represent partici-pation in any rich sense: the views of consumers or 'consumer values' are only one more set of data to feed into the decision-making processes of policy-makers, managers, and health professionals. Yet this concern with research-ing, or consulting about, the preferences and values of relevant populations is undoubtedly the most developed and most prominent form of 'community involvement' in health policy. There is another parallel I want to draw between participation at the individual and social levels. I would want to argue that, in general, the call for, and ethical case for, greater transfers of power from policy-makers to 'the public' runs up against the same problems of practicability and defensibility. That is, although many people's views can influence decisions and a number of people can, to some extent, be party to decisions only specific people are directly accountable for the decisions made. And these systems of accountability run in a number of sometimes conflicting directions—there is no 'straight line' between decision-makers and the public. I will come back to these parallels later but I also need to acknowledge the possible differences between the two levels of participation.

We might say that patients in doctor–patient meetings are only contributing to decisions about their own lives and treatments whereas a community consulted about community priorities are contributing to decisions about other people's lives and treatments. The latter seems to raise extra problems of legitimacy, the legitimacy of making choices for others. That is, the former does not raise these problems if we have in mind something like Mill's 'harm principle' (Mill, 1948), and we take the focus of the individual doctor–patient encounter to be patient-centred, with the doctor acting as an informed agent of the patient and the partnership making 'self-regarding' choices about patient change. But on closer inspection this difference between individual and community participation seems to be more a matter of degree than a matter of kind. As I have already mentioned the doctor is not, or not entirely, an agent of the patient, nor can the effects of the 'doctor–patient' choices be practically insulated from the wider community. Individual choices affect communities just as community choices affect individuals. There are, I think, some ethical distinctions to be made here, but they are not clear-cut.

Policy-makers may look to public involvement in decision-making for three things: to deepen their evidence base, to extend the democratic legitimacy of their decisions, or to strengthen the appearance of these things. This last (public relations) function is worth highlighting because it often provides a powerful motive for talking up public involvement on the other two grounds, and these may be foregrounded more in theory than in practice. Also this public-relations role should not always be dismissed as merely cynical or ethically irrelevant: in public life not only doing but being seen to do the right thing has a place. Nonetheless the principal justifications for public involvement is the same as for shared decision-making in one-to-one encounters: because better decisions will be made by respecting the community's knowledge, values, and preferences, and, many would add, because people are intrinsically deserving of the respect reflected in involvement. To these instrumental arguments and the intrinsic rationale of respect for persons can be added, in the collective sphere, the values of democracy. That is, if we aspire to a society of free and equal persons we must seek mechanisms by which individuals can have as equal a say as possible in shaping the social and material environments in which they live.

When expressed in this broad-brush fashion public involvement makes a strong ethical claim, and it would be foolish to dismiss its value and potential for improving healthcare. But in practice there are, I suggest, good reasons to be sceptical about both its epistemological and ethical bases unless its application is carefully qualified. The degree of public involvement can be presented as a spectrum (what Arnstein, 1971, labels a 'ladder of citizen participation'— from 'manipulation to therapy to informing to consultation to placation to partnership to delegated power to citizen control'). The key dimensions of this spectrum are an increase in information-sharing, an increase in decision-makers' responsiveness, and finally, an increase in involvement in making decisions. Each of these is a dimension of community empowerment and each of them is championed as part of the ethical transformation of healthcare. Why be cautious about them? I will look at each of these dimensions in turn.

(i) Transparency

There is, it seems to me, comparatively little reason to be sceptical about the principle of greater transparency in health policy. Opening the information base of decisions and the decision-making processes to scrutiny (allowing for confidentiality constraints) would seem likely to enhance the quality of decisions and serves as one mechanism for policy-makers to address their accountability to the public. This is perhaps the strongest plank in the spectrum of shifts summarized above and I will not say much more about it here. However, it is also worth noting that the way in which transparency policies are interpreted and enacted in practice may not bear much critical examination. In practice there may be a tendency to replace secrecy with a public relations driven access to carefully selected, and sometimes even misleading, 'facts and figures'. This is a good example of the potential slippage between the ethics of principle and the ethics of practice. The value of transparency policies depends, as with all else, ultimately upon what can be realized in practice, not just upon arguments of principle.

(ii) Responsiveness

In some sense decision-makers have to be responsive to the beliefs, values, and preferences of the public if they are even to do their job. Public values, in general and in detail, provide the rationale for policies and part of the evidence base for decisions. Unless we have some conception of what kinds of social 'harms' matter to people (e.g. traffic congestion, domestic violence) and the ways in which these things are impacting on people's lives we lack the proper basis for developing public-health policies. Even needs assessments for clinical-health services require evidence about the subjective experience of illnesses and their effects on families and communities—morbidity statistics alone are inadequate. But when are public values 'evidence', what is it that makes them worth noting, and what kinds of 'values' should be taken into account?

That these things are problematic should be clear. Most people would presumably not want health policies to be shaped by racist and sexist preferences. We would expect that these kinds of values would be 'filtered out' of the process somehow. Public values necessarily have to be mediated through other social processes, and we expect that these processes serve amongst other things as a filtration system. We might, for example, suggest that only 'internal preferences' should be taken as relevant, and that 'external preferences' should be discounted (Dworkin, 1977). That is, we should take notice of what individuals value for themselves but ignore their views about what would be better for other people or how health-related goods should be distributed. We might further take the view that individuals' judgements about what states of affairs they would find valuable should be respected when they relate to the 'ends' of health policy but should be treated with considerable caution when they relate to specific policies or strategies for achieving these ends. The idea behind this being that their personal knowledge makes them well equipped (although not infallible) to come to conclusions about the former but not the latter where technical expertise, of one kind or another, seems relevant. In other words we could try to adopt a model of public consultation in which views based upon prejudice, partiality, ignorance, or misunderstandings are ignored. But this stripped-down model faces two major problems:

First, whatever its potential merits, it is barely a model of public consultation. It boils down to the collection of evidence about individuals' subjective evaluation of actual or hypothetical states of health. This is precisely the sort of data which health economists collect in order to assess the costs and benefits of certain courses of action. This is better seen as enhancing the information base of decision-makers than as consultation. Second, there are notorious methodological problems both with interpreting and using such data which many health economists are only too ready to admit. For instance, how are we to handle the fact that certain groups of the population may, perhaps because of low expectations, consistently estimate their health status as 'better' than external indicators suggest (Wiseman, 1999). But, even more critically, what are we to do with such data? Unless there was near universal consistency in the subjective evaluation of possible health states we necessarily risk applying judgements based upon majority or average perceptions to population subgroups who do not share these evaluations.

This is not to deny that it is better to base decisions on consideration of these sorts of data, only to emphasize that this is not an unproblematic 'exact science'. Normative judgements are built into health-economic analyses, and these normative judgements do not emerge simply from the data nor from their aggregation by health economists; they are embedded in the construction and use of the data (Berg, 2001). This is merely one example of the way in which assumptions about health-related goods, as discussed in the last chapter, pervade the health-policy field.

One possible way forward is to look to public values to inform these normative judgements. The arena in which this has happened most commonly is priority setting. Suppose a health authority has to decide how to weight the resources and effort it attaches to prevention or therapy and/ or to different kinds of medical treatments, and/ or to the care of neonates compared to the elderly, etc. Faced with the overwhelming complexity of these judgements, the recognition that the underlying choices fall outside the domain of professional or technical expertise, and their first-order public interest importance, then policy-makers might, quite sensibly, turn to public opinion as a relevant source of judgement. Here the relationship between policy-makers and the public has moved on. The public is still not being treated as parties to the final health-policy decisions but their values are 'being respected' and taken into account in the process (Nord (1999) for example). But, as the famous Oregon experiment and many other community priority-setting initiatives have shown, this sort of exercise simply moves the underlying problem a step further back. There is still the need to interpret and apply the normative judgements made by members of the public, and, once again, this involves further normative judgements which transcend those articulated in the process of consultation. For example, if a health service is supposedly based upon a principle of equal access for equal need, what is to be done if the weight of public judgement suggests priorities which undermine this principle (Doyal, 1998)? If we move outside the priority-setting debates similar, and equally serious, concerns arise. Should, for example, widespread public resistance to forms of 'cloning' be heeded? And, if so, is this regardless of the basis of this resistance? Suppose it could be shown through careful social research that for the most part this resistance was based upon entirely false beliefs about the nature of the proposed cloning, or generalized anxieties about doctors 'playing God', would that make any difference? In short, when should public values be listened to and when should they be challenged?

(iii) Democratic involvement

There are, therefore, two contrasting dangers facing the extension of public consultation. On the one hand public consultation can be used to provide a superficial legitimacy to decisions which managers and policy-makers feel bound to make on independent grounds. This is often the suspicion in the priority-setting arena. Everyone then apparently shares the responsibility, for example for the non-availability of certain services, even though, in the end, the public's views play little role in the final decisions. On the other hand there is the danger of populism (Pateman, 1970). That is of policy-makers choosing to respond to that which is popular in situations where they have independent grounds for discounting the popular position, e.g. because it is based on misunderstandings, because it damages the interests of minorities, because, more generally, it conflicts with principles otherwise regarded as fundamental. The responsiveness of public policy-makers has to steer a course between these two dangers. And exactly the same balance has to be struck in projects which do not merely talk up consultation and responsiveness but which actually play up the role of the public as decision-makers in order to enhance the democratic basis of health policy.

These dilemmas are not easily resolved but one part of the answer involves moving towards more sophisticated conceptions of democracy. This requires, at a minimum, making a distinction between indirect and direct forms of democracy, and striking a balance between them. As well as making use of this distinction it is also essential to distinguish between the different facets of public participation in health policy: (a) agenda-setting, (b) deliberation, (c) decision-making, and (d) execution (Gutmann and Thompson, 1996). My remarks up to now have been largely sceptical about an unrestricted role for direct participation in (c) and (d) because of the need both to define lines of accountability and to protect the space for independently established grounds and parameters. But there is no good reason to rule out indirect democratic mechanisms in relation to (c) and (d), and there are good reasons to extend direct democratic participation in (a) and (b). I will say a little about each of these in turn.

Given that policy-making in healthcare should attach weight to certain basic ethical principles (such as respect for persons) and that particular health systems will have certain specifiable founding principles (such as equal access for equal need)[2] then democratic accountability includes putting accountable public representatives in place to ensure these principles are respected and to scrutinize the ways in which they are interpreted and weighed in practice. Similarly, whilst decision-making cannot be reduced to the application of scientific and technical expertise there is a public-interest need to ensure that knowledge claims are based upon the standards relevant

---

[2] These embodied values are, of course, likely to carry broad support from the relevant population. However, to argue that they are themselves legitimated democratically can be to beg the question of the relationship between ethical principles and democracy.

to the knowledge domain invoked. These independent grounds for decision-making—let us say 'ethics' and 'knowledge'—are not somehow 'against' democratic will. Provided they are subject to democratic scrutiny and public deliberation, they could equally well be presented as an expression of democratic will. Focusing on these independent grounds gives rise to the question of whether health professionals, or other relevant experts, have some kind of 'special role' so far as many-to-many relationships in health are concerned. In some cases this seems straightforwardly to be the case, i.e. some individuals (e.g. Chief Medical Officers) are appointed to authoritative, and relatively powerful, social positions on the basis of their relevant expertise and experience. Their degree of influence and special responsibilities in relation to the public good are closely linked to the networks of accountabilities which define their roles. But these public offices should not form the basis for generalization, in each case a claim for some degree of special influence on the part of health professionals has somehow to be earned and collectively authorized. The one exception to this, I would suggest, that gives a potentially special public role to all health professionals is an obligation to share their expertise in ways which enable more effective participation by others, i.e. some kind of health-education role (where health education is understood broadly). I discuss this role further in Chapter 10.

The difficulties of relying upon more direct democracy for decision-making can also be seen by reflecting on the remarks of Lomas (1997: 105): 'in our role as taxpayer we may oppose increased funding, whilst in our role of patient we may demand new and expensive services although in our role as local citizen we ...'

Members of the public are simply not required to be consistent in their decision-making, whereas their accountable representatives, whether appointed experts or democratically elected, are. Decisions have to be practically coherent with each other if they are to be realizable as well as cohering with the framing principles of the system in question. However, as the tradition of work on deliberative democracy (e.g. Gutmann and Thompson, 1996) shows, there is much more to democracy than simply making decisions, especially given the severely attenuated decision-making mechanisms, often voting, typically available. The richness of the agenda, its responsiveness to different interests and perceptions, the breadth of reasoning and evidence, and the quality of argument and public scrutiny can be strengthened through processes of open discussion and debate. As a result of all of these things it is likely that better decisions will be made and that such decisions which have, in a number of senses, more democratic authorization. This is analogous to the core advantages of shared decision-making in one-to-one encounters.

Hence although I have generally wanted to raise doubts about making reference to 'democracy' in health policy as if it were a panacea, I would not only stress the ethical importance of certain democratic forms but also the scope for their practical implementation. Perhaps the best example here is the most widely cited account of how to conduct and appraise a collective process of priority setting—the 'accountability for reasonableness' framework of Daniels and Sabin (1998). This framework requires that priority-setting decisions are made: (1) using reasons which 'fair minded' people would agree are relevant and appropriate to the specific context, (2) in a way that makes the rationales used transparent, (3) in a way that can be challenged, and (4) in ways that are underpinned by regulation which protects these criteria. But the real power of this framework is not just that it represents an articulation of principles (principles which embody a version, albeit a circumscribed version, of a democratic deliberative process) but that it is designed to be, and has been, practically implemented and evaluated (Martin and Singer, 2003).

Recognizing the role of deliberative conceptions of democracy is also a move from emphasizing sheer responsiveness towards emphasizing the quality of the reasoning behind decisions. Here again the importance of independent grounds, i.e. grounds other than 'what people want', is acknowledged. We do not simply need to discover 'what people want' but also the basis and legitimacy of their claims upon one another. We do not simply wish to disseminate power so as to try and equalize levels of influence upon decisions, rather we wish to make better, more defensible, decisions. In other words we need to look for mechanisms by which to qualify and complement expert authority with democratic authority. The alternative is simply to replace the power of the expert with the power of the majority, an exchange that may well leave the individual significantly worse off.

Conclusion

There are, to conclude, many reasons to lend support to the calls for patient and community empowerment. Democratic influence over health can and should be extended so as to correct the dangers of over-concentration of power, and so as to treat patients and citizens with due respect. But there are innumerable problems that arise from the processes of empowerment if they are not anchored in a consideration of other values and in realistic systems of accountability. What is more there are some fundamental tensions between patient empowerment and community empowerment. The public at large, as citizens of the health polity, should have some say in shaping and regulating the institutional regimes of healthcare. But these democratically authorized regimes will, in turn, shape the potential opportunities for, and constraints upon, patient empowerment. The limits of patient power are set, to some extent, by the reasoned preferences of the public. In specific health polities the relative influence of individuals and populations will be mediated by the political philosophy informing the health system and the respective institutional regimes. In all health polities this will, on occasions, put the patient as patient in conflict with the patient as citizen. The former will wish to interpret the obligations of health professionals in ways that the latter rejects.

One of the themes I will pursue later in the book is the need for the institutional regimes of healthcare to balance together personal and public conceptions of health-related goods. This balancing act can be presented as a conflict between clinicians and public-health specialists. It can, as I will go on to discuss, equally well be presented as a conflict between the person-centred face of health professionals and the population-centred face of health-service managers. But coinciding with and reinforcing these conflicts is the conflict between the legitimate claims to influence of the individual patient on the one hand and the public on the other.

Just as is the case with the health goods discussed in the last chapter, then, the cluster of values related to calls for more participation need first, to be carefully distinguished from one another and second, to be balanced against competing goods and considerations. Furthermore we have to look beyond the abstract arguments in support of greater participation and to closely consider the practical possibilities of realizing participation. What are the real-world possibilities for embodying and enacting participation? The lessons of healthcare-technology assessment have to be extended to healthcare ethics. In the end it is not the effectiveness of interventions under conditions of academic research that matters but their practical efficacy in use. The same applies to the principles of healthcare ethics. Ethicists are well placed to demonstrate the grounds to support participation and also the grounds for limiting the scope of participation, where needed, to protect other ends. But ethicists, like the public, do not have to achieve the 'practical balances' here. The shift in emphasis from expert authority towards democratic authority can be presented as an attempt to moderate undue forms of power. But it cannot be realistically presented as some kind of transcendence of power relations. Building the social authority behind health-policy decision-making is a good thing, but it is a good thing which can itself only be achieved through systems of power relations and through imperfect practical settlements within them. This is why a deliberative ethics needs to incorporate a critical ethics. The social field of health policy is partly constituted by myths and simplifications about 'partnership', 'empowerment', 'democracy', and so on. Healthcare ethicists must not be seduced by these kind (or any other kind) of value labels because what is done in these terms may not be for the best all things considered, indeed may not even be what is on the label.

PART 2

Health-Policy Ethics

4

Health Promotion in the Good Society

In this part of the book I want to raise, and respond to, some questions of 'health-policy ethics'. In the following two chapters I will look at questions relating to health inequalities and health-related responsibilities respectively. In this chapter I introduce health-policy ethics by exploring the nature and ethics of health promotion. Here I am using 'health promotion' to pick out a complex (and internally contested) movement in health policy which, roughly speaking, seeks to reorient health policy around disease prevention or community health improvement. (I will elaborate on this account below but I should perhaps say at once that the expression 'movement' is in some respects too concrete and cohesive; it may be better to speak of an ill-defined cluster of reforming discourses which have become to varying degrees influential in health policy and care.) Although the emphasis of this chapter is on the ethics of health promotion, my major concern is to highlight the implications of the issues reviewed for the theory and practice of healthcare ethics when it shifts from a clinical to a more societal focus. I will begin with some generalizations about health promotion broadly conceived and by identifying, indeed exaggerating, some of the distinctiveness of health-promotion ethics. As I go on I will qualify this account and draw out some of the more fundamental continuities between health promotion and more conventional healthcare.

The language of health promotion clearly owes much to the nineteenth-century public-health tradition and its twentieth-century transformations including the (partly incorporated and partly oppositional) development of models of health education. An awareness of this history is necessary if we want to understand the specific forms and orientations of work done in the name of health promotion. But it is also important to see that the very idea of health promotion is inherent in the opening up of the time-space continuum in healthcare. Once we see health in the context of the whole causal nexus of events and processes we can 'zoom out' from healthcare interactions to all of the possible determinants of health and illness. And once we are in the habit of thinking about the 'outcomes' of healthcare interventions, we are enabled to start thinking about the potential 'health outcomes' of any and every kind of social intervention. This is the essence of health promotion. It is a movement which seeks to turn our knowledge of the determinants of health into action for health.[1]

Introducing the Nature and Ethics of Health Promotion

I am suggesting that the idea of health promotion is a kind of logically necessary development in the historical evolution of healthcare. The different historical faces of health promotion emerge in the space between established patterns of healthcare and the logical possibility of 'universal' health promotion. I will illustrate this process briefly.

Both private and public hygiene practices reach back through all recorded history and are central to the tradition of public health. Diseases can, to some extent, be 'kept at bay' by clean bodies, foods, and environment. Public-health science was founded on the progressive extension of this principle based upon a growing understanding of the natural history of 'infective agents' along with the development of mechanisms for their control such as the purification of water supplies and vaccination. All of these disease-

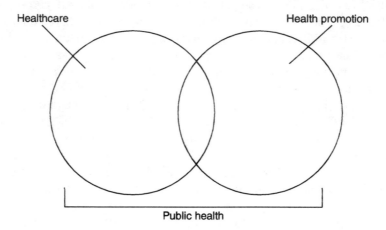

Fig. 2.

[1] In this chapter I will sometimes use the term 'health promotion' in this very general sense and sometimes in more specified ways. One of the issues is when to reflect conventional usage (which varies of course) and when to be more stipulative. This problem also arises with the term 'public health'—some of the conventional uses of 'public health' restrict it to a narrow domain, e.g. to population-oriented preventive medicine, whereas I want to use it in a very broad sense— perhaps a rather overstretched sense—to encompass the entire field of both healthcare and health promotion. The distinction between health promotion and public health in the senses adopted here, therefore, is that the former aims principally at health whereas the latter's aims include all of the aims of healthcare and health policy.

prevention mechanisms rest upon biological and physical sciences but in many cases they also depend upon the 'recruitment' of the population and hence the incorporation of educational and/or policing approaches into public health. In this way the 'technologies' of public health expand and extend across the physical and social sphere, and increasingly draw upon the social as well as the natural sciences. In other words there is a multiplication of the potential means of health promotion. Through the twentieth century this multiplication is further multiplied by advances in our understanding of the determinants of changing patterns of disease. The focus of public-health science broadens out from the control of environmental hazards and 'infective agents' to encompass both people's lifestyles and the underlying social and economic structures. The overall result of these moves is an all-encompassing frame of reference, in which any point in the causal nexus becomes a potential node for health interventions and health promotion becomes a universal possibility.

The process summarized above relates to the universalization of the means of health promotion. But the history of health promotion includes another, distinct but overlapping, dimension of diffusion which completes the 'totalizing' process; namely the frequent elision of health with welfare or well-being. I will postpone further discussion of these elisions for now, the point is simply to note that in much of the policy rhetoric of health promotion there has been a lack of differentiation concerning the ends of health promotion. (Sometimes this is for understandable reasons which I will return to later, i.e. that welfare and well-being are, in various respects, themselves part of the causal nexus underpinning health.) These elisions mean, in their most careless manifestations, that the promotion of health is simply fudged with the promotion of well-being. To promote health is to build a society in which everyone lives together harmoniously and leads fulfilling and flourishing lives.

The diffusion of means and the diffusion of ends taken together can therefore, by degrees, transform preventive medicine into a kind of utopian project. Given the necessary knowledge base and improved technologies of health promotion perhaps we can engineer a good society in which each person's suffering is minimized and happiness is optimized? Of course I am not asserting that this sort of vague neo-utopian thinking is confined to the health-promotion movement. Nor do I wish to condemn utopian models out of hand: here I take their value to be an open question. I am merely wishing to indicate how and why neo-utopianism often lies in the background of health promotion. Sometimes, indeed, it is in the foreground. For example, the WHO 'Health for All by the year 2000' strategy is a well-known example of health promotion where neo-utopian elements came to the fore. The strategy came to be associated not only with the need to improve health universally but also, for understandable reasons, with a staggeringly wide range of targets which included reduction in international conflict and civil wars.

The distinctiveness of health-promotion ethics, therefore, relates in part to the apparent boundlessness of health promotion. Who are the agents responsible for health promotion and whose health are they supposed to be promoting? Is everyone responsible for promoting everyone's health? Apart from those people working in public health, or in posts with a named health-promotion function, it is difficult to know who else to include in, or exclude from, the category of 'health promoters'. If we think about the range of potential opportunities for promoting health then we might be inclined to include everyone. However, if we ask who has not only the relevant expertise but also the ethical legitimacy to promote other people's health we may be inclined to exclude almost everyone, perhaps even many who work in public health. The more we move away from one-to-one health promotion encounters, e.g. a doctor counselling a patient about dietary changes, the more these problems of expertise and legitimacy come to the fore for three very good reasons.

First, the longer and more complex the causal chains involved the harder it is to attain reliable knowledge of the effects of interventions. In so far as these interventions involve changes to social or cultural systems as well as to physical systems the problem is compounded because of the notorious problem of attaining predictive validity in the social sciences. Second, more 'long distance' health-promotion interventions will inevitably produce more complex systems of 'side effects' which are not only difficult to predict but also difficult to evaluate. Given the complex causal and constitutive links between aspects of health, welfare, and well-being already noted then such evaluations, as well as the predictions they rest upon, have to be multidimensional. Third, and perhaps most important of all, whereas healthcare practices are composed within an elaborate professional ethic including systems for 'permissions' and role-specific obligations there does not appear to be any equivalent process of 'ethical licensing' for health promotion. Prima facie it is difficult to distinguish health promotion from well-meaning interference in other people's lives.

Some of the other general ethical challenges facing population health promotion have been mentioned in earlier chapters. For example, as well as the question of whether something analogous to informed choice is meaningful or possible in population contexts, there are the problems of weighing individual claims against population claims, and the difficulties of understanding the idea of, or force of, population-related goods including overarching social ends such as efficiency, equity, or solidarity. In short, in addition to questions of expertise and legitimacy, questions of paternalism, utilitarianism, and social justice are always likely to be prominent in population-oriented health-promotion ethics. The classic dilemmas in public-health medicine provide clear examples: the coercion of individuals to control the spread of an infectious disease and the use of social incentives or disincentives to promote compliance with a screening programme even for those who will not benefit from it themselves. To a large extent all the dilemmas in population-oriented health-promotion ethics will be analogous to these ones.

Of course not all health promotion is, on the surface, population-oriented. Indeed, arguably the most widespread penetration of health-promotion discourse has been in the contexts of clinical healthcare where it refers to the introduction of a longer-term health maintenance, health enhancement, or disease-prevention orientation into professional–client encounters. Here the issues of health-promotion ethics interact with those of clinical ethics. There are two competing ways of thinking about these interactions. We can see the conventional structures of clinical ethics and professional–client relations as somehow anchoring health promotion in an ethical 'safe harbour'. Or we can see the different orientations of health promotion as potentially disrupting and undermining these conventional structures. (How we should think about this issue is, in some respects, a central problem for this book, and I will return to it more explicitly in later chapters.)

I have, thus far, presented health promotion as an extremely diffuse movement which incorporates preventive medicine and neo-utopianism, and both population and one-to-one approaches. The common rationale, which holds these things together, is the emphasis on the full range of means for the production of 'health outcomes' (somehow understood). This range obviously includes very different kinds of things, and in order to discuss the ethics of health promotion in any more depth one has to focus in on particular forms and examples of health promotion. I will do a little of this in the following section, although my interest in doing so is more methodological than substantive. That is, I am less interested in whether such and such an example of health promotion is ethically justifiable than in the implications of examples from health promotion for healthcare ethics and health policy. Also I will keep one eye on the more generic issues that I have just introduced. The movement from preventive medicine towards utopianism brings to light something of critical ethical relevance. Health promotion 'invades' more and more domains of our lives, and reconfigures them as domains of public health. In the process the categories and values associated with these domains are also reconfigured; we can conceive of this, in sociological shorthand, as an extension of the 'medicalization' of life. The expression 'healthism' is also used sometimes to capture the risks of this reconfiguration and revaluation of social life.

The Framing of Health-Promotion Ethics

From what has been said above it should be clear that health-promotion ethics represents an 'opening out', or even in some respects a dissolution of, the comparatively circumscribed concerns of clinical healthcare ethics. In the rest of this chapter I will more systematically sketch out the contours of this broadening agenda through the exploration of a few examples; starting from within a relatively narrow focus and moving, so to speak, outwards. This process also illustrates the importance of the 'framing' of healthcare ethics: what is seen as crucial to a problem depends both upon the contexts in which it takes place and also the way the problem is described, including those aspects of the contexts we stress. (This question of framing is one I return to in several places, in particular in Chapter 6 when I discuss 'the agenda problem' and in Chapter 11 where I pull together the methodological conclusions of the book.)

To begin with a routine scenario from a clinical setting: imagine a patient (Peter or P), who smokes cigarettes, eats an unbalanced diet, and takes virtually no exercise, and who goes to his doctor having recovered from a series of relatively minor but debilitating coughs and colds and says in effect, 'What can I do to prevent this from happening to me in the future? I would really value your help and support on this.' The doctor (Debbie or D) then faces some fairly familiar, and potentially uncontentious, questions of professional ethics. Suppose D decides to concentrate on encouraging P to stop smoking and begins by checking that P wants to stop, what then ought D to do? D might apply (although not necessarily self-consciously) both 'rule-based' and 'consequence-based' styles of ethical thinking, asking (a) what is it ethically permissible for me to do here; are there certain courses of action which are simply unacceptable from an ethical point of view; or are there certain things I am ethically required to do? and (b) what would be the outcome of a range of different actions, which potential outcomes are good, bad, or better or worse, what would be an adequately good and/or an ideal outcome?[2] Much of this is unlikely to be self-conscious or cognitively exacting because the scenario is one in which the doctor's professional habits, routines,

---

[2] The relative importance of each of these dimensions of ethical thought, and the extent to which they are either meaningful or defensible as accounts of ethics independently of one another, is the subject of a great volume of ethical theory and debate which I will leave aside here. Of course there is a price to pay for leaving these things aside. In particular I am forced to use expressions which 'fudge' together different possible readings. For example, in talking about the possibility of certain courses of action being 'simply unacceptable', I have chosen not to make a distinction between certain actions being 'intrinsically unacceptable', irrespective of their consequences, because they breach some non-consequentialist account of ethical foundations, and their being 'obviously unacceptable', where the ethical judgement made seems clear-cut for whatever reason. This latter is consistent with a consequentialist account in those cases, for example, where the likely harm is very great and the possible benefits are negligible.

and repertoires will be activated and because P and D are enacting widely understood social roles within well-defined social institutions and settings. (The relevance of the latter can be seen by imagining instead that this encounter takes place at a birthday party and that D happens to be P's next-door neighbour.) But, supposing that the reasoning was made explicit, the major ethical concerns can be easily simmarized: how far is the D 'authorized' to act here; how confident is D as to the desirability of the ends of her actions; and what 'forms of influence' is it acceptable for her to bring to bear on P?

We can call the interest in 'rules' or 'consequences' (or indeed 'virtues' as the third member of a fairly standard classification of ethical perspectives) the *axiological dimensions* of health-promotion ethics. My working assumption is that each of these three dimensions picks out something of relevance to the ethical evaluation of health promotion. What I take to be major questions of substance such as those about authorization, the evaluation of ends, and the defensibility of means can be called the *substantive dimensions* of health-promotion ethics. My working assumption being that these different substantive dimensions can be approached with more or less emphasis on each of the axiological dimensions. In short, I take the dimensions of health-promotion ethics to be essentially the same as those for healthcare ethics as a whole. In the case under consideration, for example, it makes little ethical difference whether D is considering a preventive intervention or if D is facing a question of treating P for a disease. One difference, however, which is worth briefly signalling, is that in this instance the nature of the personal influence that D exercises over P (does D educate, persuade, threaten, or reward P? etc.) is highlighted as the focal point of P's actions. This factor is of equal relevance in therapeutic transactions but is sometimes pushed into the background because some drug, surgical intervention, or other technique is centre stage. What we see as the 'mode and medium' of possible transactions between D and P—the sorts of actions in question, whether they involve overt technology, the extent to which they are 'aimed' directly at P's body or at P's beliefs or other mental states, or at P's cultural or physical environment—is one element of what I mean by the framing of health-promotion ethics. To ask about frames is to ask 'How is the phenomenon under ethical scrutiny constructed?'

In the case of P and D, as in other cases, the phenomenon is both socially and conceptually circumscribed. It takes place, assuming it to be a real case, in a defined social context which has a physical, institutional and discursive constitution.[3] And the ethical matter in question is described with specific

---

[3] Of course there will not be only one valid characterization of that context, rather there will be multiple accounts, to some extent emphasizing different features of the context and to some extent competing with one another. But I am assuming some variant of a realist position in this idea of social framing; I am assuming that there is, as it were, *one* social context which can be described within a broader or narrower focus and in various ways.

emphases. For example, in the scenario above the doctor–patient consultation takes place, let us suppose, in a specific primary healthcare setting, the norms of which are 'second nature' to both D and P, and the scenario is described in a way that insulates the encounter from a range of wider ethical considerations. D is clear that P wishes to stop smoking and that smoking has an almost entirely adverse effect on P and P's family's health and well-being ('almost' because the satisfaction of smoking cannot be discounted), a consideration of the wider social costs and consequences of P's smoking adds little of relevance, all that remains are concerns about acceptable forms of influence. Is it acceptable to use intimidating tactics, or to exaggerate the risks to P's family, or to set up some highly intrusive model of surveillance, and so on?

We can contrast this case with one in which P is not D's patient but is simply a resident within the Health Authority area in which D is a doctor. The Health Authority have, for some reason arising from their public-health strategy, established a community smoking cessation task force and D is a member of it. D and her colleagues are then faced with a set of challenges about what to do, the choice of which raises ethical questions. The obvious differences are: 1.The question of authorization is obscured: what are the Authority's reasons, and whose reasons are they? 2. The benefits and costs of smoking have to be considered through a social rather than an individual lens: in practice this means (i) all smokers, whether or not they would prefer to stop, fall within consideration, and (ii) the health effects of all 'passive smoking' and the social acceptability of smoking in public places become relevant. 3. The range of possible settings and actions which the Authority might consider using multiplies because they are focusing on smoking behaviour in the spaces within a geographical area, not merely the smoking behaviour of individuals.

The social frame of this new scenario is more dispersed. It roughly coincides with the Health Authority as an area and as a form of governance. We are forced to consider the legitimacy of the Authority, and the proper scope of its legitimacy. The conceptual framing of our ethical analysis shifts, in broad terms, from the discourses of professional ethics to the discourses of political authority and power. We might, for instance, make out a plausible argument along the following lines: the state and its local agencies have a widely accepted and democratically endorsed obligation to protect the health of citizens. The fulfilment of this obligation may also have other economic and social advantages. If smoking is a threat to the health of the population then reasonable measures by authorities to encourage non-smoking can be justified. This might include the enforcement of non-smoking in public places to protect non-smokers, and might also include certain moderate threats or inducements to persuade smokers to stop. These smoking-cessation measures can be justified on public-health grounds and possibly also on more paternalistic grounds, if the harm of, and the addictive nature of, smoking is taken into account.[4]

Things get more complex still if we imagine that D is a member of a more general 'Health Improvement' panel that is advising the Authority on a broad agenda of health-related issues. As well as doctors and other health professionals the panel has as members a wide range of environmental and social-care professionals and representatives of local companies and voluntary organizations. They are, on this occasion, debating 'safe drinking' and the regulations surrounding the sale and consumption of alcohol within the town. It is easy to see that the range of possible perspectives is considerable. The evidence base for the causation of diseases (such as cirrhosis of the liver, cancers, stroke, and coronary heart disease) by alcohol consumption—at least from more than moderate levels of drinking—has to be considered. There are concerns about the incidence of drink-driving offences and the risks to public safety. Alcohol-related violence is an important factor to many. Some are concerned about groups of young people congregating noisily around shops that sell alcohol. Local bars and public houses wish to stress their role as community centres and the social capital that they therefore support. The Health Improvement panel may also consider a wide range of possible interventions. They might concentate mainly upon educational initiatives, they may consider tightening or altering regulations on sale or consumption (perhaps outlaw the drinking of alcohol in the town centre outside of licensed premises), or they might use economic incentives to try and alter people's drinking patterns, for example, pressing for cross subsidy between alcoholic and non-alcoholic drinks. Each of these forms of influence could be subjected to ethical scrutiny, and the varying degrees of coerciveness involved in these measures is certainly one factor of ethical relevance.[5]

In these circumstances what is D's role? The lines between medical and social agendas have become very blurred and it is not clear where the boundaries of her expertise and professional authority fall. Similarly it is not clear what has happened to her relationship with, and obligations to, P and her other patients. D might be party to measures which impede P's ability to pursue his preferred lifestyle without any potential health benefits for P. The complications of this broader scenario arise from the causal and constitutive relationships between health, welfare, and well-being mentioned above. The panel is discussing both health issues and issues to do with the broad quality of life of the local community. There is no easy or conclusive

---

[4] These sorts of arguments are explicated in full, and analysed in detail, in Goodin's (1998) *No Smoking–The Ethical Issues.*

[5] As Wikler (1978) demonstrates in his exemplary paper on the ethics of health promotion.

way of separating these things out from one another. Violence, for example, can be seen as something which is itself intrinsically undesirable, or as something which mars the quality of social life generally, or as a factor which contributes to the oppression of women and children, and it can also be seen as a cause of (and at times a consequence of) mental or physical ill-health.[6] Here it is possible to emphasize either the discourses of preventive healthcare or the discourses of social order. Alcohol-related violence, for example, can be seen as a product of ill-health 'by definition' simply by labelling alcoholism or alcohol abuse as 'health problems'.

As D moves from a professional–client role to a health-policy or public-policy role she moves into a different, and less well-defined, 'ethical space'. As I indicated in the last chapter the institutions and discourses of healthcare do not only construct health agendas but also construct ethical agendas, roles, and relationships. One aspect of these processes of social construction is the creation of some relatively well-defined social spaces, healthcare institutions for example, where roles, obligations, and entitlements are relatively 'laid down'. The actors involved do not necessarily carry these agendas and expectations into other social spaces. And, as I have been illustrating here, many other social and ethical spaces are relatively ill-defined. For certain purposes we can undertake ethical analysis wholly within limited institutional frameworks. However, I want to suggest that this only makes sense if it is done self-consciously as itself a limited form of ethical analysis. A full ethical analysis must take into account the interrelationships between spaces, including the ways in which particular institutional norms and ethical agendas are created.

From Healthcare Ethics to Social Ethics

As the social frame of health promotion becomes more dispersed and diffused the issues of health-promotion ethics become less well defined. Indeed, it becomes increasingly contentious to call them questions of health-promotion ethics at all, as they bear less resemblance to issues in healthcare ethics and more resemblance to issues in social ethics or political philosophy. The questions of authorization are about social and political authority, the questions about ends relate to every conceivable kind of good, and questions about means mushroom to include every area of social and public policy. All of this raises second-order but fundamentally important ethical questions about health promotion: 'When ought we to analyse social

---

[6] There are some circumstances where violence can be reasonably understood as a consequence of physical ill-health. For example, men who are in the process of adjustment to serious spinal injuries are frequently violent with their nursing staff.

and political issues as issues of "health promotion"; what are the ends served by treating something as an issue of health-promotion ethics; and when and where is it defensible to describe issues in this way?' There are issues where this description seems relatively non-contentious, such as debates about water flouridation. There are other issues where it is arguable that the name of 'health' has been hijacked in the pursuit of other agendas. This kind of hijacking can work in very different directions. An environmental group may use population health-protection arguments to try and curb the activities of a local corporation even though evidence of possible harm relates more to biodiversity than directly to human health. A political authority may restrict mildly subversive forms of recreation or assembly on the basis of the risks they pose to health.

There are certain 'markers' which enable us to identify questions as falling within the arena of healthcare. Childhood vaccination programmes (which I discuss in Chapter 11), even though they are a public-health measure, have all these markers: (a) they are directed at the management of disease, (b) they involve healthcare technology, i.e. technology which interacts with the body on the basis of clinical sciences, (c) they are undertaken by a health professional, and (d) they are undertaken in a recognized healthcare institution or setting such as a primary-healthcare clinic, or by someone attached to such an institution. Ethical questions raised by interventions which have these characteristics, including questions about the organization and resourcing of such interventions, are unequivocally questions of healthcare ethics. To the extent that one or more of these markers is missing the questions become less easily insulated from other areas of social life. These are the markers through which the social and conceptual framing of healthcare is achieved, and the partial absence of which leads to the relatively weaker framing of health promotion and health-promotion ethics. The rhetorical and political significance of the framing of healthcare, and the related ethical importance of treating health as a special good, was discussed in Chapter 2. I need to underline once more that this framing or separation of healthcare from other social processes should probably only be seen as a plausible myth which relies upon questionable assumptions about the relative autonomy and neutrality of clinical science and professional authority and on 'thin' conceptions of health.

The mythic nature of this neat separation of healthcare from broader social life is highlighted by a number of other issues in healthcare ethics, for example: (a) the cultural and religious construction of attitudes to the body (body parts, sexuality, dead bodies) which can be embedded not only in the attitudes of individual patients and health professionals but also in institutional norms, most obviously in faith-based institutions; (b) the conspicuous overlap between questions of healthcare-resource allocation and broader questions of politics—questions about the relative importance of healthcare in society, and about both distributive justice and identity politics; (c) the growth of technologies which are used in medical settings but which are not straightforwardly disease-management technologies but either concerned with bodily 'enhancement' or with social concerns such as shyness. The totalizing perspective of the health-promotion movement crystallizes and heightens this recognition of the imperfect distinction between healthcare and general social life. Health promotion takes disease management and health improvement beyond healthcare settings and health-professional arenas into the public sphere, and it sometimes does so in a way that obscures any distinction between health and social ends.

The case of D, as part of a medical consultation, encouraging P to stop smoking falls squarely within the frame of healthcare. No technology may be used in the process, although it may be in the form of nicotine substitutes for example, but the other markers are clearly present. It is thus easy to treat P's smoking as a discrete disease-inducing practice, and to see smoking-cessation techniques as analogous to disease treatment or preventive vaccination, i.e. as techniques for intervening in aetiological chains of causation. At a societal level this enables us to see smoking as a 'health risk' which we can study epidemiologically, like any other cause of disease, and which we can develop social technologies to defeat. Of course in so doing we must also take some notice of the fact that smoking is a social practice which people may, to varying degrees, choose and value. This becomes clearer still when we turn to alcohol consumption where there is simply no good reason to equate the drinking of alcohol with 'disease causation' (except perhaps if we are talking about high levels of drinking), and where the social practices surrounding drinking have a range of other well-known 'good' and 'bad' effects on the quality of individual and social life. When it comes to campaigns about 'wise', 'sensible', or 'safe' drinking we are no longer operating purely within the confines of healthcare. We are clearly in the midst of broader cultural, moral, and political concerns. The same applies to campaigns about safe foods, safe sex, or safe roads, and indeed just about every other possible social issue. Because health promotion is a universal possibility almost anything can have a health-related face, and conversely all health-promotion issues have faces other than health promotion.

This migration of 'medical thinking' from clinical to societal agendas can, unless we are very careful, add up to an ideological masking of complexity. The 'ideology' here has three faces—a slide from health protection to health promotion; the construction of 'disease analogues', and a narrow framing of descriptive and evaluative models. First, there is a near collapse of the distinction between health protection and health promotion; between on the one hand negative health effects as a side-constraint on social action, and on the other hand positive health outcomes as an end of action. If all agents and agencies are recruited to the business of health promotion then the obligation not to cause disease is thereby transformed into an obligation to prevent it. Second, this 'translation' is combined with the translation of 'health risk' into 'disease analogues' so that the whole of the social world can be seen through the lens of disease management. This is the apotheosis of the medical model and of medicalization. The case of teenage pregnancy, introduced in Chapter 2, and governments' drives to 'tackle teenage pregnancy,'[7] will serve as an example. There are some significant risks to the health of very young mothers and to their babies but these are only a comparatively small part of the range of social 'harms' conjured up by the policy imperative of teenage-pregnancy reduction. As was said in Chapter 2 health-related policies cannot be separated neatly from other kinds of policies, and they need to be evaluated in the light of their complete set of justifications and effects. One of these effects, I would suggest, is the treatment of teenage pregnancy, in at least some of the accompanying policy formulations and analyses, as a disease analogue framed within the discourses of preventive healthcare. This takes the well-known problem of the medicalization of pregnancy to a new level. It is not only that pregnancy is seen through the lens of the medical risks associated with it. It is also that certain pregnancies, regardless of whether or not they are 'wanted' or 'physically healthy' pregnancies, are seen in themselves as the object of preventive medicine; are, in effect, seen as 'disorders'.

This example will also serve to illustrate the third face of the potential ideology of health promotion, the narrow framing of descriptive and evaluative models, and the relevance of this ideology to healthcare ethics. In summary, the compound effects of what is sometimes labelled as 'medical model' thinking can close off crucial ethical issues and lead to a dangerous partial sightedness. The danger is that if we think in terms of disease analogues and reduce our responses to complex social phenomena to those which are designed for disease management then (a) we will crucially restrict the range of, and distort the nature of, phenomena we are responding to and (b) we will cause harms and wrongs which are invisible within the frame of reference we are using. This is the ethical importance of the discussion of what I have called conceptual framing and, in particular, of applying narrow conceptual frames to so to speak 'broad' phenomena. Both aspects of this Procrustean tendency are worth signalling, i.e. both its descriptive/explanatory aspect and its evaluative/normative aspect. And it is also worth stressing that this problem applies as much to the relatively 'simple' health risks such

---

[7] In the UK 'Tackling Teenage Pregnancy' the focus of has been substantial programme of policies and initiatives (Department of Health, 2000).

as smoking as it does to those that are obviously complex social matters such as teenage pregnancy. Work in health-promotion research can very easily transfer an approach to causal inference from areas of clinical research where it is fitting to other areas where it is inappropriate or, at best, unreasonably 'stretched'. For example, the modelling of the causal relations between cigarette-smoking practices and certain diseases is very different from the modelling of the causal relations between the socio-cultural-economic field and smoking practices. Given the very long and complex causal chains that apply in the latter instance we need to be very cautious about whether and when we have the knowledge base to successfully 'intervene' in them. (This question was mentioned at the beginning of this chapter and is discussed again, in more depth, in the next chapter.) The second aspect relates to the reduction of social goods/harms to clinical goods/harms, a reduction that creates, reinforces and applies an ideology of disease management to fields which need more differentiated and subtle analyses. Thus if we 'know' that, because of its causal role in disease processes, cigarette smoking is always and everywhere bad, and our interpretation of evidence and construction of strategy is entirely shaped by this mindset we will simply ignore important facets of reality and we are likely to ride roughshod over people's cultures, identities, and preferences.

Given the complexities rehearsed here I suggest it is important to see health-promotion ethics as multifaceted. To make progress with issues in health-promotion ethics academics or practitioners need to be able to work with the same axiological and substantive dimensions of ethical thinking that they bring to clinical professional ethics but they need to be able to apply them to a much larger set of potential interventions and do so in broader and more contested fields. When health-promotion interventions are narrowly and strongly framed by the institutions of healthcare then they closely resemble clinical professional ethics. Here the specific professional obligations of the health promoter, and the relationship between the health promoter and their client, are highlighted. With broader and weaker framing two other major sets of concerns become prominent. First, are the many other substantive ethical disputes and judgements about both health-related and non-health matters that fill the social fields within which health promoters operate. For example, in the case of teenage pregnancy, disputes about sexuality, sexual maturity, contraception, or abortion; or, in the case of food safety or nutrition, disputes about environmental sustainability or animal welfare. Second, are the many questions about power and legitimation, i.e. in addition to the familiar questions about professional authority we are faced with broader questions, on whose behalf are health promoters acting and on what bases can they justify interventions in the name of health? A full ethical analysis of health promotion would, therefore, range across these three facets. But, as I have wanted to stress throughout, the same is true for clinical healthcare ethics; it is only the latter's strong institutional framing that sometimes obscures this point.

Even sticking close to professional–client ethics there are useful lessons from health promotion for healthcare ethics more generally. As I have indicated health-promotion interventions draw attention to factors which are sometimes not foregrounded, such as the different *'forms of influence'* in use in health settings. Alastair Campbell (1990) has, for example, explored the defensibility of persuasive tactics in health promotion and the apparent preferability of education to persuasion. His analysis raises questions about simplistic intuitions in this area and warns against generalizations of the 'education-good, persuasion-bad' variety. He shows that in practice we have to set these notions in specific contexts. How important is the end in view?; is education a realistic ideal here?; what are the (opposing) persuasive forces already faced by the client?; is the 'persuasion' an open appeal to the client's autonomous judgement, or more covert and manipulative? There are no easy answers about the acceptability of persuasion. Health professionals working in real-world settings cannot achieve entirely clean hands as regards influencing their clients. That is to say they may arguably be more culpable if they aim for the 'educational high ground' and forgo some honest persuasion.

Health promotion also highlights the *collective nature* of healthcare. This is because it is often conducted by teams or through large-scale programmes and because it is typically informed by population ends. This clearly sets the professional–client relationship in the context of the system-population, and highlights the issue of how far the 'partial' and personal nature of the former should be accommodated to the impartial, impersonal concerns of the latter. But, once more, health promotion is not fundamentally different in this regard. Nowadays all healthcare systems are organized around these individual–collective balances being achieved through various models and regimes of management. (I discuss the ideas of health professional 'partiality' and regimes of management in Part 3 of the book.)

Finally, health promotion makes conspicuous *the overlap between health and politics* and, in relation to the power of the health agenda itself, the dangers of the medicalization of social life. But these same issues penetrate all of healthcare. There is no point simply analysing whether health professionals are going about their business in ethically acceptable or desirable ways. We also need to ask whether this 'business', considered in the light of the full breadth of its effects, reorients personal and social values and priorities in ways which are acceptable or desirable. Healthism, used in the pejorative sense I mentioned earlier, signals the over emphasis on certain goods at the expense of others.

Social Technology or Political Philosophy?

There is, however, a danger in placing emphasis upon medicalization or healthism that health promotion is analysed only as a means of hijacking or distorting broader social concerns. Health is an important good, even if only one amongst many, and the impact of broader social, economic, and political factors on the experience of, and distribution of, health is unquestionably a matter of fundamental practical and ethical importance. The tradition of public-health science and medicine has also conclusively demonstrated the substantial population benefits that can be achieved by applying our knowledge of the determinants of health into strategies for the pursuit of health. Furthermore much of this work can quite appropriately be couched in the language of preventive medicine. It is possible to frame public-health goals in the language of health and illness, for example by aiming for a reduction in the incidence of heart disease or the cancers, without rolling these goals into other social agendas.[8] Health is one of the few plausible candidates for the position of a relatively value-neutral 'primary good' in conditions of value pluralism. If it is possible to organize our affairs so as to reduce the incidence of illness then there is a very powerful prima facie case for doing so: people who are less ill, other things being equal, are fairly uncontroversially better off, and, again other things being equal, a world with more people better off is a better world. Obviously these assertions have to be qualified by the consideration of health-promotion ethics (Is the conception of health in use really a good in certain instances? Are the methods used acceptable? Are the side effects of health promotion acceptable?). But, it might be argued, we had better treat health-promotion ethics as a side constraint on the worthwhile endeavour of health promotion rather than as a course of wholesale critique and deconstruction.

From this perspective health promotion can be seen as a form of social technology that uses the full range of social-science understanding to extend public health. This perspective on the social world has illuminated people's experience of health and illness in ways that have fundamental ethical relevance, two aspects of which form the axes for the following two chapters. First, it has shown the striking correlations between socio-economic status and health status: poorer people generally live shorter and less healthy lives. Second, it has highlighted the causation of illness (in ourselves or in others) through human agency. There are now countless studies which contribute to our understanding of both inequalities in health and to the role of agency as a

---

[8] Of course this does not mean that the means recommended or used do not intersect with other social agendas and other goods—this would be impossible—only that the ends can be analytically separated out.

determinant of health. The fact that we are in a position to have informed debates on the ethical issues of equity in, and responsibility for, health has been facilitated by the commitment to a more detached scientific rigour in the study of public health.

Yet even whilst paying homage to the scientific achievements of health promotion and public health, and even whilst acknowledging the merit of trying to insulate the scientific analyses from the ethical disputes, we have to keep in mind the fact that health-promotion sciences are necessarily value-laden. All accounts of the public health, however scrupulously constructed, are, as I argued in Chapters 1 and 2, inevitably normative accounts. They are formed from notions of what matters, they involve concepts and measures which count certain things more than others, and they are presented with particular emphases. In the health-promotion literature this normativity is partly recognized and addressed in the debates about approaches and models (discussed further in Chapter 10): How much should health promotion focus directly upon disease prevention or upon other aspects of welfare or well-being? How far should explanations and interventions centre on individual behaviour change or upon broader structural factors? How far should research or interventions be designed to address inequalities in health? In practice, in other words, questions about such things as responsibility or equity are interwoven with the scientific and technological questions.

Another way of approaching this point is to ask, if we see health promotion as a social technology, who operates the technology? This takes us back to the problem of authorization and legitimacy. It is no good merely asking 'what can be done' to promote health, we are also forced to ask 'who is, practically and ethically, in a position to do something?'. In this sense the matter of agency and responsibility is unavoidable, and in this sense it is plausible to see issues of health-promotion ethics as, at base, about political philosophy. Of course sometimes the questions of political philosophy will be very much in the background. That facet of health-promotion ethics which is about health-professional ethics, particularly within strongly framed healthcare settings, raises many issues that deserve attention in their own right and which are not, in the main, issues of political philosophy. The doctor who is engaged in patient counselling or education, or in delivering screening or vaccination programmes to her patients, for example, must consider their professional obligations, and be sensitive to the various harms and benefits flowing to their patients from their actions. It is equally necessary to ask about the doctors' ethical comportment and character, and their engagement with a professional 'community of practice' (Wenger, 1998) including relevant social norms and institutional guidelines. But lying behind all of these things are the actual and potential values of the health polity in which health professionals work. A doctor's role and authority, and the scope and limits of her activities, is defined by social, legal, and political structures. The social and political construction of professional ethics, as introduced in Chapter 3, is clear enough from clinical medicine. Doctors are not allowed to provide any treatments they wish, even where they might judge these to be in the interests of their patients. Social limits are set with regard to controversial interventions such as abortions or physician-assisted suicide, or because of socially authoritative judgements about the safety or efficacy of treatments or, in many circumstances, for reasons of collective priority setting. More generally the conduct of health professionals, and the realm of permissible forms of professional behaviour, is socially defined. We can, therefore, ask 'how *ought* these things to be determined and defined; or in other words what *ought* to be the shape of the health polity?' Once again the relevance and importance of these questions about the social and political context becomes more obvious in relation to health promotion, where health professionals and others are working in the heart of the public sphere. Some of the examples discussed in this chapter, such as alcohol or teenage-pregnancy policies, are obviously bound up with questions of political philosophy. For example, they raise questions about political authority, the place of democracy or forms of expertise in social decision-making, the distinction between the public and private spheres or public and private goods, and the legitimacy of the state or state agencies in constraining or influencing individual people's options or choices.

This can be illustrated by returning to the 'least contentious' case featuring D and P as a professional and client meeting in a health centre. If P wants to change his lifestyle then D no doubt ought to offer help and support in this direction. However, D may well think that she also ought to direct some of her efforts to the broader determinants of P's 'lifestyle choices', perhaps local environments and policies or broader commercial pressures. Also D might reflect on the factors that inform her own choices about what combination of approaches to use and what tactics to deploy directly with P. How, she could ask, do political, economic, and commercial pressures bear upon her own reasoning and choices? Are performance indicators in place that, for example, work to reinforce an individualist rather than a more collective approach to health promotion? How does her budget help shape the choice of approach? Do incentives from pharmaceutical companies influence her reasoning about the use of nicotine substitutes? The shift in emphasis from health care to health promotion is often described as a move 'upstream' (McKinlay, 2001), a move towards the consideration of 'earlier' causes, a move back in time to before 'the damage gets done', to before the options are closed down. An analogous move is needed in healthcare ethics. If we are ethically serious we need not only to ask 'Given these options what ought we to do?', but also to ask 'From where do these options arise, and how might they be changed for the better?'

The Facets of Health-Policy Ethics

The three major facets of health-policy ethics mentioned above—those questions that are akin to clinical ethics, questions about the other matters in the social field of action and those about background systems of power and legitimation—might be seen heuristically as professional ethics, 'citizen ethics', and political ethics. These three facets can, to some extent, be considered independently but are in reality interdependent. Here I am using the notion of 'citizen ethics' to capture questions that I referred to earlier as the substantive ethical concerns which fill the social fields in which health promoters work, e.g. concerns about animal welfare, sexuality, etc., and also to indicate that these are questions 'for everyone'. In so far as the idea of citizens can be used to point up that which all persons have in common they are questions of universal relevance. On the other hand the differences in social identity and social position between individuals mean that they are questions which can be approached from a multitude of vantage points. For individual citizens questions of health-promotion ethics include the questions about how individuals weigh the relative importance of health to other goods in their own lives, the extent to which they assume responsibility for their own health or for the health of others, and the ways in which they justify their own actions in these regards. Analogous questions, relating to the axiological and substantive dimensions of health promotion, can be asked from the point of view of both political ethics and professional ethics. In addition these three perspectives have to be understood in relation to one another. And it is not simply that professional ethics are 'nested' within political ethics in the way that I have indicated in this section. Rather each perspective can be used to ask questions about the other two.

What this means, I would argue, is that the ethical evaluation of health-promotion interventions, whether education campaigns or tax incentives or whatever, require a compound analysis. The conduct of the health promoter requires ethical scrutiny and this facet can be treated as if it was relatively autonomous. But a definitive assessment of the ethical defensibility of health-promotion interventions will normally be dependent upon a parallel analysis of the context of the intervention including the surrounding social ethics and health polity. An example from penal ethics might make these somewhat abstract points seem clearer. The actions of a prison officer seizing cannabis from the possession of a prisoner can be assessed so to speak both 'internally' and 'externally'. The internal ethical assessment would begin from the professional norms within which the officer is working: have these been applied accurately, sensitively, fairly? The external assessment would question these norms. Is it right that prison officers should have these sorts of powers? Is it right for individuals or the state to treat cannabis differently from tobacco? The assessments are only relatively autonomous because (a) in a social climate where penal attitudes towards cannabis have been generally relaxed,[9] for example, it could be argued that prison officers might have an obligation to interpret or apply their own norms more liberally and (b) prison officers can reasonably argue that their own experiences and standards are ethically relevant to determining wider social and political norms.

The complementarity of what I have just called internal and external evaluation will be a background theme for the remainder of the book. This means combining an interest in conduct within ethical spaces with an interest in the construction of ethical spaces. How can social roles and corresponding sets of obligations be conceptually and practically defined in ways that do justice to the public good, the interests of citizens, and the particular contributions of healthcare professionals? In the following two chapters I will approach this question by asking, in very general terms, about the distribution of health-related goods and obligations.

[9] For example, in recent UK drugs policy and more particularly in an experiment in the London borough of Lambeth.

5

The Distribution of Health and Healthcare

Introducing Health Inequalities

Arguably the most important ethical implication of the diffusion of the health agenda is the growth in salience of health inequalities. Taking a broad social perspective on health opens up the consideration of patterns of determinants and patterns of health experiences. An epidemiological lens requires that we do not only ask questions about the population as a whole but also ask questions about the differential experiences of groups within the population. For example, if the people in city A suffer much higher levels of life-threatening diseases than their near neighbours in superficially similar city B we want to know why that is, and lying behind that interest is an interest in what might be done to bring the health experiences of city A closer to the levels currently experienced in city B. There are two possible concerns, working separately or together, here. First, is the notion that the gap between A and B indicates the existence of unrealized health potential in A, and more health being a good thing, other things being equal, we should be concerned about this unrealized potential. Second, is a concern that there is something prima facie unfair in people's health experiences, including their chances of being seriously ill or dying earlier, being 'determined' by their postal address. Very often these concerns are expressed almost as 'intuitions', as if their basis was clear-cut and unproblematic. In this chapter I want to consider these concerns with health inequalities in a little more depth, not merely to ask 'Are these concerns justifiable?'—which I will argue they are—but also to consider: (i) What they might entail in practice, i.e. 'What would a more equal health polity have to aim at?' and (ii) How far should health or public policy be led by a concern with equity where this comes into conflict with other relevant values? In the first part of the chapter I will set out my reasons for thinking that health inequalities are ethically important. As I proceed I will place more emphasis on the problems of interpreting the implications of this ethical significance.

I will begin with a science fiction type example or thought experiment. (I do not want to rehearse the arguments for and against this sort of methodology, but I will note that I do not see this example as being decisive, simply as being indicative.) Imagine a chemical compound, 'Equipush' or EP, which has 'magical' properties. If added to the water supply of Scotland (let us suppose it is entirely specific to Scotland, having been developed by Scottish-regarding aliens) it does the following: (a) it lowers the disease and death rates of the (up to that point) least well 90 per cent of the population to the rates of the other 10 per cent; (b) it has no effects on the relative distribution of disease and death within the 90 per cent; (c) it has absolutely no side effects whatsoever, including no effects on other aspects of welfare and well-being.[1] In these (albeit absurd) circumstances what advice should a public-health panel give to the Scottish First Minister about putting EP in the water supply? It seems clear to me that because of its staggering health benefits EP should be used, but I need to acknowledge that there are reasonable arguments to be made on both sides. Possible arguments against are: 1. Many people may have an understandable reluctance to rely upon mysterious 'magic', and prefer to leave the management of their own well-being to less effective but more transparent human knowledge. 2. Some people will not want to have their water supplies 'tampered with' in this way, and, despite the absolute guarantees of safety, bitterly resent being denied the choice. 3. Some of the people who are 'benefited' may not want to live longer lives and, if asked, would prefer a 'natural' life-span. 4. The EP treatment has the effect of reducing the diversity of human experience and diversity is, in itself, a good thing. 5. To the extent that the longer and healthier lives of the 10 per cent is something which is deserved by them (on some account) EP may undermine the proper place of desert, and undercut related incentives to live healthier lives. I will ignore the first objection and treat it as if it were overridden by the suspension of disbelief involved in the thought experiment itself.

Each of the other four objections deserves consideration, but none of them, I would suggest, is strong enough to curtail the use of EP. The diversity point is the weakest because there is no reason to suppose that the overall diversity of human life is going to be significantly affected by the single fact that people will have more similar patterns of ill-health between social groups. But it is worth noting because it highlights the fact that any single value, however thin, can at least in principle be set against the pursuit of greater equality. The denial of choice is, of course, important but there are a number of moves which can be made against it such as: (a) underlining the fact that all of the water supplies are already 'tampered with' for reasons of health protection, so it is unclear why the line should be drawn at EP, especially given the absolute guarantee of its safety; (b) ensuring that there is at least some degree of public decision-making and

---

[1] This last condition makes the example not only practically impossible but also, I think, logically impossible. We might imagine that the economic effects of EP cancelled each other out, less treatment on the one hand but longer-term provision on the other, but the broader interactions between health experiences and life experiences mean that these things are internally related not externally related.

democratic legitimacy by, for example, balloting the population. It seems likely that the vast majority would be in favour of using EP; (c) if possible ensuring alternative supplies of bottled drinking water for those who continue to object 'on principle'. Similarly the fact that some people may not want to live longer or be healthier is ethically important but can be better dealt with by making alternative provision for these people (either alternative supplies of water or even arrangements such as physician-assisted suicide) rather than by denying the benefits to those who do. The argument from desert is harder to deal with. I will need to come back to it again later. But here I can simply mention two worries we might have about making this argument decisive against the use of EP. First, we would have to attach a lot of weight to the importance of desert if it is to override the huge benefit of many people's lives being greatly improved with regard to health. Second, we would need to be confident that our attributions of desert were entirely valid. These judgements are both epidemiologically and ethically complex, and not least because there is a counter-case to be made out for the deserving claims of the least well-off. Because I cannot imagine overcoming these two worries in this case I would advocate the use of EP. (We could also weaken this concern about desert by reworking the scenario so that EP also has some beneficial effect on the health of the 10 per cent, so that it narrows the 'health gap' rather than eliminating it—see below.)

What are the implications of this imaginary example for real-world efforts to address health inequalities? What happens if we replace the magical technology of EP with the existing social technology of HP (health promo-tion)? I would argue that the same considerations still have relevance—respecting people's choices and wants, possible side effects, and questions of desert—and it is clear, I think, that they all bite much deeper in the case of HP than with EP. However, I would also argue that there is a very strong *prima facie* case for attaching priority to addressing health inequalities which these various considerations and possible objections have to overcome.

What are health inequalities and why do they matter?

Health inequalities are now a prominent feature of health-policy agendas, but it is important not to talk about health inequalities as if they were natural phenomena like floods or hurricanes, or perhaps a type of disease epidemic. It is not merely that we should avoid the medicalization of social phenomena but also that we need to keep in mind the contested nature, and to some degree the constructed nature, of health inequalities. I say this not because I have any doubts about the reality or ethical importance of inequalities in health but because I think there is plenty of room for doubt about exactly what aspects of inequality to focus on, and of the implications of so doing.

Up to now I have been referring to statistical variations in mortality and morbidity between different population groups, but the phrase 'health inequalities' could refer to a number of other things. For example: variations in levels of access to health systems and healthcare (which may of course be a cause or effect of variations in disease patterns); variations in the opportunities for participation in healthcare decision-making; variations in the experience of ill-health (some groups of people may experience ill-health in better environments, with more personal or professional support, etc.); variations in the levels of social respect or stigmatization that are attached to different health-related conditions, social settings, or identities. There are many ways in which social organization and relations can fail to embody equal consideration—inequality is not one-dimensional. I will return to the plural nature of health inequalities later in the chapter. For the most part I will concentrate on what is sometimes known as the 'social-class gradient' in health: the significant correlations between socio-economic status and health status as measured in death and disease statistics. Also in most of what I say I will ignore the question of what underlies these correlations, and in particular how they relate to the plural nature of inequality. That is, it is not just that people can be unequal in a range of different ways,[2] each of which directly affects well-being and the distribution of well-being, it is that there are various possible causal mechanisms that may link these different dimensions of hierarchy to the distribution of health experiences understood more narrowly (disease and death). The 'social-class gradient' is not necessarily, or purely, about the links between material deprivation and ill-health, it might equally well represent links between a lack of social power and ill-health.

Whatever the mechanisms that explain it there is an overwhelming body of research that shows that as the overall health experience of people in broadly affluent developed nations has risen the social-class gradient has stayed in place.[3] The advantages of relative affluence in terms of longer and healthier lives have not been shared equally but have disproportionately benefited those people who are better off in other ways, i.e. in blunt terms those who have better housing, better education, better jobs, more money, status, and power. Of course there is not a universal correlation between these things and better health, but if you want to make statistical predictions about the length of people's lives these factors will provide very useful indicators for your predictions.

[2] For example, in the ways in which Bourdieu (1986) analyses as arising from the differential ownership of a range of different *forms* of 'capital' (e.g. economic, cultural, social, and symbolic).

[3] Many would say that the gradient has become steeper, that is that the health gap between the richer and poorer sections of such populations has widened. This claim, however, depends upon how you conceptualize the relationship between two different gaps in two different historical periods, crudely between (a) 'worse off' and 'better off' in former times and (b) 'better off' and 'better off still' in later times.

I will take it that this is a true account of things and ignore 'flat-earthers' and others who would fundamentally call it into question. However, I cannot move from this stance to the conclusion that health inequalities have the sort of ethical significance that many people, especially many public-health specialists, give them. Without being a flat-earther you could perfectly well accept the statistical significance of the correlation between socio-economic and health status but deny the correlation ethical significance. 'This', you might say, 'is simply the way things are. The better-off always have been and always will be better of in multiple respects, living longer is simply one of these. This is no one's doing, and no one is to blame for it, it is just a fact.' The thinking behind these sorts of remarks does not represent a 'straw' position. It closely echoes the kind of thinking manifest in a number of neoliberal and 'New Right' positions articulated by academics and politicians in the last quarter of the twentieth century. This thinking tends to deny the relevance of 'end-state' patterns of distribution to the assessment of social justice, favouring instead a conception of justice as fair procedures for cooperation and exchange between free agents. The distributive patterns are more or less discounted because: (a) patterns are abstractions and do not in themselves affect the well-being of any one individual, (b) patterns are not the outcome of any individual's actions and so no individual can be held responsible for having caused them, and (c) any measures which were designed to change these patterns are liable not only to be ineffective but also to significantly undermine individual freedom and the fruits of freedom. Different thinkers might place relatively greater or lesser emphasis on each of these three discounting factors, but considered together they constitute some basis for scepticism about the ethical significance of health inequalities.

It is, I would argue, important to concede some ground to the sceptic. The fact that there are variations in conditions or experiences between people is not in itself of ethical significance. It would, for example, be possible to map variations within a population in the number of face freckles, or in the number of television channels available to people but to discount these things because they do not represent variations in well-being or sufficiently important indicators of well-being. Or it would be possible to map major variations in the quality of life due to the uneven distribution of certain serious diseases but question the ethical significance of these variations because the diseases in question affect people entirely because of some uncontrollable 'natural lottery'.[4] Finally it would be possible to identify some variations in health that, for whatever reason, had prima facie ethical significance but then argue that

---

[4] Although, of course, others may well argue that even if the causes of these disease variations are uncontrollable their effects on life opportunities create ethically salient inequalities which are in themselves, to some degree, rectifiable.

the harms or the wrongs that would be caused by attempting to rectify these inequalities would be of far greater ethical import than those represented by the initial variations. But I suggest that it is a gross mistake to add these considerations together and imagine that the combination amounts to a knock-down sceptical argument against the health-inequalities agenda. For a start the final point is not an argument against the ethical significance of health inequalities. On the contrary it concedes that health inequalities can have significance but then asserts that the attention we give to them also requires us to balance this significance against other ethical concerns. The real force of the sceptical position relies on the first two points. To the extent that variations in health status are seen as one set of variations amongst many naturally occurring variations, and to the extent that they are seen either as not especially indicative of variations in well-being, or as having causes or effects which fall outside the scope of human agency, then the sceptical position succeeds. But neither of these conditions is very plausible. Indeed in both cases the initial plausibility seems to be in the opposite direction. Although it is a mistake to equate health status with well-being, health is a widely recognized component of well-being, in many ways a determinant of broader well-being, and at least sometimes a relevant indicator of well-being. Similarly the entire history of medicine and all of the work that has gone into public-health initiatives and the organization of healthcare systems is predicated on evidence that variations in the experiences of ill-health are at least amenable to human action.

The ethical significance of health inequalities was summarized in the example of EP discussed above. Health inequalities seem to suggest unrealized health potential on the part of the 'less healthy' groups and/ or they suggest the existence of some unfairness or injustice in the distribution of health protection. In brief they indicate either unnecessary harms or potential wrongs. The positive ethical case for addressing health inequalities can be put in these terms: to the extent that we can find ethically permissible methods for organizing our affairs so as to achieve greater equality in opportunity for good health we should do so, otherwise we are colluding in the processes that condemn some people, for reasons outside their control, to lives of lower welfare and reduced opportunity. The relevance of 'reasons outside their control' depends upon accepting something like Dworkin's 'choice–circumstance' distinction (2001), i.e. that those inequalities in access to goods (including health goods) that result simply from the circumstances that individuals happen to find themselves in and are not a byproduct of their freely made choices are ethically problematic because they undercut equal opportunity (I will leave aside the question of the ethical acceptability of 'choice-produced' inequalities). The ethical relevance of equal opportunity is already accepted by most people in relation to the accessibility of basic healthcare. Advocates of welfare systems have typically asserted the need to achieve greater equality of access to medical care, and done so on the basis of the importance of equal opportunity to welfare. These arguments have also been theorized by a number of philosophers (e.g. Plant *et al.*, 1980; Doyal and Gough, 1986) who have highlighted the importance of equal opportunity to basic needs satisfaction as a precondition of the conditions for a liberal polity, and hence as the corollary of the enforcement of the obligations of citizens. Plant, for example, has questioned the coherence of calls for free and equal participation in society without a corresponding collective emphasis upon securing the conditions for participation (Plant and Barry, 1990). Most famously Daniels (1985) has extended Rawls's analysis of social justice to include a consideration of health as a 'special good', i.e. as a good which is relevant to the possibility of securing a 'normal opportunity range' for all citizens. Daniels's argument, therefore, does not support calls for equal access to any and all kinds of healthcare, but does attach a fundamental ethical importance to securing fair access to basic healthcare. Whether or not we believe these sorts of arguments work philosophically the direction they point in coincides with the direction of compassion. It is difficult to imagine most people standing by comfortably whilst their neighbours who were dying or seriously ill were visibly being denied healthcare.

Tackling Health Inequalities

The problem with accepting these sorts of arguments is that their implications are potentially very radical indeed. Once we understand that the main determinant of health status and of inequalities in health is not healthcare but the general conditions of social life then these arguments, about the importance of equal opportunity for health, push us towards root and branch reform of society. If less well-off groups of people live shorter and more diseased lives it matters little whether this is caused by lower access to medical care or by greater exposure to disease determinants. As long as these differential experiences are amenable to modification then the argument from equality of opportunity has at least prima facie relevance. Of course these manifestations of health inequalities may be much less visible than those caused by a lack of access to care. A number of people dropping dead from heart attacks that might have been preventable, for example, may not cause a scandal but as well as representing preventable harm they may also represent an example of unequal health opportunities. From the standpoint of equity the lack of visible 'neediness' or 'unfairness' is arguably irrelevant. What matters is that certain people have had less chance than others to live longer healthier lives, and enjoy the resulting benefits, for reasons outside their control.

Once again I would like to stress that I am persuaded by these arguments about the ethical importance of addressing health inequalities. I do so because I now wish to say something about the many obstacles facing those of us who are impressed by these arguments. The cumulative effect of these obstacles may seem a sufficient basis for abandoning this focus but I do not think they are. These obstacles include (a) a lack of clarity about the ends of tackling health inequalities, (b) a high degree of indeterminacy about the knowledge base for tackling health inequalities, and (c) the ethical costs of measures to tackle health inequalities including the conflicts between health outcomes on the one hand and other health and non-health-related goods on the other.

What are we aiming at? In order to decide on criteria for success in reducing health inequalities we need a clear account of precisely what makes such inequalities ethically undesirable. For example, we need to be able to answer this question: are preventable inequalities in health bad in themselves regard-less of what causes them or what their consequences are, or are they only bad to the extent that they are (a) caused by unfair institutions or practices and/ or (b) lead to unfair distributions of well-being? There are a number of reasonable positions here and which one we favour will depend upon our theories of ethics and justice, and our account of the relations between health and well-being. I will not pretend to answer these questions here although I will make some further remarks about them below. The point is that we need to be cautious about stipulating the goals here, and of course the nature and intensity of any strategy will depend upon the formulation of the goals.

Another crucial aspect of goal indeterminacy, only alluded to thus far, is the question of how the 'health gap' ought to be closed. A gap between 'better-off' subpopulation A and 'worse-off' subpopulation B can, in prin-ciple, be closed by raising the health of B, lowering the health of A, or raising the health status of both but B's by more than A's.[5] Are we aiming for simply a 'narrowing of the gap', by whatever means, or a 'raising up' of the less well-off group? This reflects an important axis of controversy in both political philosophy and practical politics. Rawls's (1972) famous defence of the 'maximin' principle (maximizing the position of the worst-off in society as one of the core principles of justice) is seemingly compatible not only with wide disparities in welfare between members of society but also with meas-ures which further widen these disparities if these measures can be defended as consistent with achieving the best absolute level of welfare for the worst-off. However, it is possible to argue that wide gaps in the distribution of welfare between social groups is in itself a bad thing. But even from this perspective the extent to which reducing this gap by measures which also

[5] Of course you could lower them both but B by less than A, but I am not treating this as a serious candidate.

have the effect of lowering the absolute standard of living of the most vulnerable members of society has to be debatable.[6] This tension between addressing relative or absolute deprivation is at the heart of all social policy and it certainly has relevance to health inequalities where it seems reasonable to claim that in conditions of affluence absolute deprivation has been dealt with more effectively than, and perhaps at the cost of, relative deprivation.

Do we know how to tackle health inequalities? This question embraces the question of whether we understand the causation of health inequalities, but is not the same as it. There is no doubt that a great deal is understood about the causation of socio-economic and other (e.g. gendered) patterns of ill-health. For this reason I will not dwell on philosophical puzzles about causal explanation here. I certainly would not want to suggest that the existence of relevant philosophical questions somehow undermines the credibility or seriousness of well-entrenched claims about the causation of health inequalities. (By way of analogy, to raise philosophical questions about the extent to which we have a definitive causal model of the relationship between cigarette smoking and lung cancer would not be the same as questioning the fact that cigarette smoking causes lung cancer, although, of course, this is how certain lobbies might like to see it.) The philosophical questions in this area are mainly questions in the philosophy of science and philosophy of social science. In a sense the problem here is not so much a lack of evidence and theory but one resulting from a proliferation of evidence and theories. Let us suppose we know that groups who are 'disadvantaged' in relation to indicators such as occupation, income, housing, education, social status, locality, etc. will generally be disadvantaged in relation to morbidity and mortality statistics. To what extent can we claim to know the causal processes at work in these cases? [7]

---

[6] In reality these debates are, of course, not conducted in such a pared-down form. They have at least two other components. First, theoretical and empirical debates about social and economic possibilities—what combinations of welfare distribution are attainable? Second, some more fine-grained discussions about conceptualizations and measures of welfare, which include, for example, discussions about the extent to which personal welfare is itself constituted by (or caused by) social equity or inequity.

[7] Here I will largely leave aside some of the complexities relating to alternative conceptions of health and health inequalities, but it is worth noting a couple of examples of the complexities arising from other possible conceptions. First, if we broaden our construct of health to include various other dimensions of human well-being then the correlation between socio-economic well-being and health becomes true, to some extent at least, by definition. We cease to deal with causal patterns and begin dealing with constitutive relationships as well. This is a general problem with more holistic conceptions of health inequalities: the more holistic we get the less we can separate out 'health' from other factors in our descriptions and explanations. Second, if we move away from expert-dominated conceptions towards lay conceptions of health we cannot simply assume the same correlation between socio-economic status and health. Seriously disadvantaged groups (such as Australian aboriginal people) often report relatively higher levels of health experience compared to their health profile as measured in morbidity and mortality statistics. This, obviously, raises the

There are very many methodological problems in providing definitive causal explanations of differential experiences of health. As is well known the range of potential determinants (genetic, environmental, cultural, life-course-related, lifestyle-related, economic, etc.) and the number of possible interactions between them is huge. Even the interrelationships between the factors mentioned above (education, occupation, income, social status, housing, locality) are extremely complex. What we are looking at is, as Graham puts it, 'an intricate web of hierarchies' which makes up socio-economic inequality (2000). Tracing out the causal pathways that flow from the strands of this web to the differential risks, susceptibilities, incidences, responses to, and experiences of, ill-health is extremely daunting.

These methodological challenges have both a 'technical' and a philosophical face. There is the technical difficulty of demonstrating the rigour of putative explanations. For example, the way in which Wilkinson has combined survey research with theories of psycho-social aetiology to explain the prevalence of health inequalities in affluent settings has been criticized by some as lacking adequate explanatory depth and rigour (see Forbes and Wainwright, 2001). But there are also even more fundamental philosophical problems in the telling of causal stories, for example: (a) how does one identify the limits and framing of causal chains, how far back in space-time does one go, and how does one recognize significant nodes in the causal nexus?; (b) in particular how does one handle human agency as a part of these causal chains; and given that agency is one causal element, whose agency should be foregrounded in the explanations proferred?[8]

If we know what causes health inequalities then we have some idea how to go about tackling them. Similarly, to the extent that there are uncertainties in our descriptions and explanations, including philosophical uncertainties about causal framing or agency, then we will be uncertain about the best way to go about reducing health inequalities. But, to repeat, questions about tackling health inequalities cannot be reduced to questions about the causation of health inequalities. Again consider the analogy with smoking and lung cancer, assuming that there is a definite causal link here, and that there are no technical, epistemological or other philosophical problems to be found in describing this link, how does this knowledge help us 'tackle' lung

---

question of how far we should attach weight to 'lay' versus 'expert' patterns of inequality. In addition it raises the question of how far we should simply accept and respect lay accounts, or how far we should treat them as something which themselves require an explanation.

[8] One widespread acknowledgement of the first issue here is found in the debate about how far 'up stream' or 'down stream' health policy should place its emphasis. One widespread acknowledgement of the second issue is the debate about striking a balance between 'empowerment' models which are premised on the possibility of agency and 'anti-victim-blaming' strategies which recognize the constraints on certain forms of agency.

cancer? Anyone who has thought about health promotion soon recognizes that 'knowledge for intervention' is different from 'knowledge for explanation'. Even in the case of smoking there are: (i) multiple potential points of intervention, e.g. the uptake of smoking, the smoking habit, the cigarette, biological, for example genetic, intervention (in principle) and (ii) problems in identifying the optimum intervention set, e.g. how much intervention should be at a structural or individual level, how far interventions should be educational or more coercive, and problems in identifying at whom interventions should be aimed (for example, politicians, industry, health professionals, everyone, all smokers, some smokers). These same problems exist in the case of health inequalities but are, of course, many times more complicated.

Here the limitations of the social sciences become all too apparent. To make judgements about the effects of the kinds of interventions which are often called for in the case of health inequalities, e.g. more redistributive taxation, investment in the infrastructure of deprived local environments, reform of benefits and so on, requires extraordinarily complex modelling. And even where this modelling may indicate effectiveness there will be a strict limit to the generalizabilty of this reading across time and space. I think it would be reasonable to claim that as things stand our knowledge about effective intervention is almost a reverse image of our knowledge of causation. The latter, despite philosophical difficulties, is substantial. The former remains relatively minimal. There is some sign of progress here however as represented by the imaginative analytical framework for public-policy assessment set out by Margaret Whitehead and colleagues (Whitehead *et al.*, 2000), but these same authors would be amongst the first to acknowledge that the dominant conceptions of what counts as rigorous evidence based claims cannot be achieved in this area. What is needed here is a more flexible notion of evidence-informed reasoning.

What are the 'ethical costs' of tackling health inequalities? Of course even if there is a prima facie ethical obligation to try and reduce health inequalities, and even if we knew how to, it would not follow that it was right to try. It is possible that there are equally telling, or more telling, sets of obligations which press in the opposite direction. These countervailing ethical pressures have been anticipated in the EP example and in other places in this part of the book. They include the full catalogue of issues in health-promotion ethics: attaining authorization, resolving contestable ends, and identifying defensible means. We can simplify these further here, for heuristic purposes, by asking about the 'opportunity costs' of tackling health inequalities. How would public policies aimed at reducing health inequalities impact on other goods? What relative priority should be attached to this end rather than other kinds of social ends?

Clearly the answers to these questions depend upon a thorough examination of the full range of potential measures. Each measure will be implicated in a range of causal lines and a cluster of goods. As was mentioned in Chapter 4 educational interventions will tend to raise fewer questions about the curtailment of freedom (although they are not neutral in this respect) than measures, say, which 'outlaw' certain lifestyle choices. In each case these measures will support or undermine ends other than the distribution of health, e.g. conceptions of informed citizenship or 'civic order'. It is possible also, and this depends upon empirical examination, that in order for a measure to have the desired effect on the *distribution* of health, and not just on the overall promotion of health, that it would have to substantially constrain the economic freedom of certain people and agencies in ways which are ethically questionable. (This is not, however, to embrace the automatic assumption that all constraints on economic freedom are bad from the point of view of either ethics or efficiency, or that redistributive taxation, for example, is a salient indicator of illegitimate violation of personal autonomy.) The various links here are 'supercomplex' (Barnett, 1994). Even from the point of view of health and healthcare the range of goods which needs to be considered is huge. This discussion has revolved around the distribution of disease and death. But it is widely understood that these are sometimes not the most important factors even in strongly framed healthcare settings. People will sometimes trade an earlier death for a management of their disease which enables better functioning. Likewise they may trade levels of functioning for gains in other aspects of their quality of life. Someone who is seriously ill, for example, needs to be able to live their life, understand what is physically happening to them, feel cared for, be helped to make sense of their changing circumstances, and participate in decisions about their care. Each of these things (and there are others) represents a good which deserves attention alongside the postponement of disease progress and death. A world in which absolute priority was attached only to these latter things would be a nightmarish one.

In addition there are the ethical complexities relating to authorization and accountability. Who, if anyone, is responsible for these things, and who is entitled to act on the basis of them? We have already seen that there is a potential place for the government, health professionals, citizens, indeed any and every agency. And if we think in terms of some supposed collective obligation here what are the social mechanisms for underpinning it, can or should it be enforced on anyone apart from, perhaps, the state? These questions are further complicated because they are bound up with philosophical puzzles about causal and ethical responsibility. As in the EP case it makes all the difference whether we see individuals as somehow 'creating and deserving' their own personal health experiences and the advantages of better health, or whether we think that social arrangements should be designed around the recognition of, and fostering of, *shared* responsibility for health. (This is the subject of the next chapter.) In any case we cannot adopt a purely technological approach to health improvement as if we were dealing with 'blind' causal chains when all of these causal chains are intertwined with forms of agency and responsibility.

What, therefore, can we conclude about the putative obligation to tackle health inequalities? It seems clear from the above that at best it is an obligation that we should approach tentatively and with some humility. Nonetheless I am wary of the temptation to forget it just because of these multifarious complications. (Many of us should probably be doubly wary because it suits those of us who are more affluent not to 'discover' these obligations.) It is possible, at least in principle, not only that some health inequalities are matters of injustice which might be rectifiable but also that some methods of rectification are broadly consistent with other good ends and are, as methods, ethically defensible. So long as this is the case health inequalities represent a sufficiently fundamental and far-reaching ethical problem to merit a high profile on the health agenda. And, it seems to me, that if we move away from this abstract consideration of a possible obligation to looking at empirical realities, and to the kinds of things such an obligation might entail in practice, its claim on our ethical imagination becomes much more, and not less, convincing. I say, 'it seems to me', because I doubt that this is the sort of thing which is amenable to argumentative demonstration alone; these issues are too interlinked with unresolved empirical questions and the ideological frameworks through which these are interpreted.[9] One of the things that I think can be drawn from the above discussion is the near impossibility of doing some kind of ethical 'cost-benefit analysis' of large-scale attempts to do 'redistributive health promotion', the costs, benefits, causal lines, and responsibilities being all too complex and contested. But if we begin with a more modest focus and ask about the health opportunities and experiences of the worst-off members of society, and what could be done to improve their health experiences, and whether these things ought to be done, then matters become more compelling. (This may, of course, mean putting the idea of 'patterns of outcomes' and the 'breadth of the gap' in the background, and concentrating more on what counts as 'absolute deprivation' in affluent societies.) First, it is clear that the most disadvantaged people typically experience multiple forms of disadvantage which undermine equal opportunities. In certain communities or social

---

[9] I do not want to assert that it is necessarily beyond demonstration, merely that it is so from my perspective as I write. Many of the empirical questions may be answerable and much of the ideological disagreement may be closed down if they were.

groups there is a high concentration of environmental risks, unemployment or insecure and poorly paid employment, inadequate housing, poorly re-sourced schooling, and low levels of access to health services or social health insurance. Second, even if we were to assume, and this is an extreme assumption, that individuals were entirely responsible for protecting the state of their health after the age of 18 (or equivalent marker of 'adult compe-tence'), the long-term impact of these first years of disadvantageous life conditions on individuals' health careers is enormous. For a start individuals brought up in certain circumstances will die earlier than they might have done because of this fact, and do so because of many factors which are susceptible to change but which are unequivocally beyond their control. Third, steps taken to ameliorate these risks to long-term health will involve the amelioration of other negative factors which generally detract from welfare and well-being. I do not want to obscure the problems associated with such steps—the possibility that such 'welfare measures' can have vari-ous negative effects or the problem of ascribing responsibility, e.g. 'who should pay?'—but I think that these three observations make a persuasive starting-point when we come to operationalizing the argument from principle.

Health as a Touchstone of Equal Consideration

Whatever we think about the case for attempting to tackle health inequalities through extensive social and health-promotion measures questions of health and social justice are inseparable. There is widespread acceptance that equal consideration in healthcare is important—one might even see this as defini-tive of ethical healthcare—and this is often interpreted as requiring emphasis upon greater equality of access to healthcare. As mentioned above these sorts of views are also supported by arguments about the foundational importance of health as a condition for equal opportunity more widely. At the main-stream social and political level these arguments have become integrated in modern health polities. In this final section I will assume that there is something in these arguments but show the need for us to collectively interrogate their implications and importance. And in concluding I will reaffirm the notion that health is, in some respects, a special good, but also somewhat reformulate the account of its special status.

As I have indicated above there is no knock-down argument for the primacy of 'disease-freedom' over other valued ends. Indeed, it is often a comparatively minor determinant of well-being. Many people would happily trade a little less disease-freedom for some more of other things, e.g. sex, money, art, friendship, and in many instances we would think them right to do so. Equally there are a number of other broadly 'foundational' goods (income, education, etc.) which are key determinants of equality of opportunity, and against which health claims have to be balanced. For these reasons I am sceptical about attaching too much weight to 'health', in this narrow sense, as a touchstone of social justice. However, if we look at 'disease freedom' in combination with the other goods served in strongly framed healthcare contexts, which I have gestured at through the label 'health goods', then the case becomes much stronger. Health goods in this sense were listed above as including, for example: the need to be able to live one's life, understanding what is physically happening, feeling cared for, being helped to make sense of one's changing circumstances, and participating in decisions about one's care. Healthcare is, in short, valuable because of 'care' as well as because of 'health', and if we wish to treat our fellow citizens with equal consideration then we need not only to consider the social distribution of health states but also the social distribution of care, concern, and support. It is this combination which, I suggest, makes the widespread intuition about the 'specialness' of health so compelling. It is not merely that we do not wish to see the health of people neglected, it is that we do not wish to see people neglected.

In fact, as I signalled earlier in the chapter, the full health-inequalities agenda is much broader than the one I have concentrated upon, indeed it is a many faceted agenda. Even if we could agree on a decisive account of the ethical importance of greater equality in health-related matters we would still have to wrestle with problems of interpreting and applying this goal in the light of this multifaceted agenda. There is, as I have indicated, a large range of relevant health-related goods to consider and balance both in principle and in practice. This challenge can be formulated in different ways. We could think of the goal in terms of an overall pattern of distributive justice: how can we underpin a fairer 'distribution' of the relevant set of health goods such as health states, knowledge, care, or participation? Policies designed to deliver greater equality with respect to one kind of good may work against equality with respect to another. (For example, as discussed in Chapter 3, policies that widen participation in decision-making can potentially lead to less equity in provision; such tensions are not inevitable but neither can we assume that equity goals are always compossible.)

Alternatively we could think of the goal as about meeting and attempting to reconcile competing conceptions of justice. Nancy Fraser, for example, distinguishes 'economic justice' from what she calls 'cultural justice' (Fraser, 1997) in order to distinguish the (sometimes competing) ethical demands of redistribution and recognition. Her account is an overarching analysis of the need to consider both (a) forms of economic deprivation, marginalization, or exploitation and (b) forms of cultural domination, non-recognition, or disrespect. This latter axis is constructed largely around the matter of respect for cultural and personal identities but it has both direct and indirect relevance to health inequalities. We can ask about how specific health policies and practices valorize certain identities rather than others, for example about modes of stereotyping and institutional discrimination in patterns of diagnosis and treatment. And we can also extend the underlying concern with respect and recognition to 'health and illness' identities, to the ways in which both the realities and taxonomies of differential health experiences elicit varying compounds of social regard, concern, and compassion.[10]

One significant implication of these plural conceptions of justice (Cribb and Gewirtz, 2002) is that they push us away from the assumption that justice is 'arbitrated and dispensed' entirely by some central agent such as the State.

If we accept, for example, that social justice demands the recognition of diverse identities and modes of association that include rather than marginalize, then we are all responsible for the promotion of social justice. For in our everyday lives we must struggle to ensure that our personal relations with others are informed by principles of social justice and the institutions in which we operate take social justice concerns seriously. (Cribb and Gewirtz, 2002: 19)

In short these plural conceptions highlight the ways that responsibility for social justice is diffused and is shared by both 'centre' and 'periphery'.

These analyses of social justice have major implications for health inequalities and health policy. In a nutshell they mean that a concern with health equity cannot and should not, as it often seems to, just focus on attaining greater equality in access to available treatments (nor even on greater equality in access to those treatments deemed to meet 'needs'), rather it must be based upon a broad-ranging interpretation of equal consideration. Here I will just stress two implications of equal consideration which are central to my account. On the one hand it means addressing the processes of care and the extent to which care is equally respectful of, and sensitive to, persons irrespective of their personal characteristics or what they are suffering from. This means tackling various kinds of institutional and individual discrimination. On the other hand it means taking steps to ensure that health opportunities are not inequitable, i.e. that large differences in people's chances of being ill in the first place are reduced as far as possible unless, and to the extent that, there are good reasons not to do so. (To put it like this puts the 'onus of proof' on those who would resist.) In practice, as I have noted, this means that there may sometimes be tensions between equality of access, equality of respect, and equality of opportunity for health. Policy-makers and practitioners will have to make choices about which to prioritize in

---

[10] Similarly we could apply a threefold model of justice as involving distributive, cultural, and also associational elements to capture interest in inequalities in participation as well as in the health-outcome goods and the processes of care and respect. (Cribb and Gewirtz, 2002)

specific sets of circumstances. For example, recent emphasis in the UK on enhancing the health opportunities of the 'socially excluded' have arguably taken some resources and attention away from the provision of certain expensive treatments, the absence of which impacts differentially on specific groups of patients. There is no reason to suppose that there is one 'ideal' system of funding and institutional arrangement that will meet all equity goals equally.

Here, as usual, there is a tendency to place attention on those aspects of equity that are the most concrete and the most measurable. Up to a point this seems wise. Access to treatment is relatively measurable and has relatively manifest and measurable effects. It is, at the same time, a publicly visible symbol of social compassion (or on some accounts social solidarity). Reducing inequalities in 'care' or reducing the extent of remediable divergence in health opportunity are, by comparison, relatively amorphous and contested notions. However, it is becoming increasingly clear that the degree of emphasis placed on access to treatments is undue. In particular the diffusion of the health agenda, and the social reflexivity that comes with it, has changed the character of the debate about access to health opportunity. Inequalities in health opportunities, and the factors which underpin them, are increasingly understood. These inequalities are becoming less invisible, more visible. Epidemiologists and health professionals have an obligation to explain these issues, including the social-class gradient in health experiences, to the wider public, and are increasingly so doing. The more this happens and the more these inequalities remain in place the more implicated we all become in their persistence. The more this happens the more the fact of diffused responsibility is driven home. Unless we have a strong account of why these inequalities cannot or should not be addressed their continuation shifts from being an unfortunate fact of life to being a clear, concrete, and well-understood sign of a lack of equal consideration and social compassion. In other words greater social reflexivity means that wider health inequalities come to play the same practical and symbolic role that inequality in access has played to date.

6

Responsibility for Health

Who is responsible for whose health? This question, like its archaic equivalent, 'Am I my brother's keeper?', indicates the two 'directions' of judgements
about responsibility. In relation to health promotion, for example, we can
ask both who the health promoters ought to be, and whose health they are,
individual or collectively, obliged to promote? More generally we can ask
about the most defensible patterns of obligations and entitlements in relation
to health-related policy and healthcare. This issue is, of course, therefore
closely bound up with the concerns of the last chapter. As we have seen
equity cannot be separated from responsibility. In so far as equity involves
responding to desert and not simply need we need an assessment of people's
responsibilities and how well they are discharged; and, the other direction,
even given some account of what equitable treatment requires we also need
an account of how the responsibility for securing equity is divided up. (In
some cases, for example, it makes little sense to somehow 'require' individual
citizens to deliver greater equality, however they may well have a duty to
press for social mechanisms which serve these ends.)

To begin with such a general, and admittedly vague, focus as the right
pattern of health-related obligations and entitlements is to ask for trouble.
This is a question that is normally asked within defined parameters of one
kind or another. Within a health polity[1] we can, for example, debate; (a)
legal and economic restrictions on business corporations on health and
safety grounds, (b) the right pattern of funding for healthcare, (c) the extent
to which individuals with certain infectious diseases can legitimately have
their freedom of movement curtailed, or (d) whether smokers should 'lose'
some of their entitlement to healthcare. Each of these questions is difficult
enough considered on its own. What is more, even if we were able to make

---

[1] As I indicated in the Preface I have chosen to limit the scope of this book to the relationship
between healthcare ethics and public-health ethics within a health polity. This choice does not
flow from, and is not meant to be indicative of, a particular ethical stance on my part. It is simply
a pragmatic strategy to circumscribe the (already large) range of issues I discuss. Nonetheless the
choice of this polity-related focus, rather than one upon global relationships, may have some
unfortunate ethical implications. I will say a little more about this later in the chapter in my
discussion of 'the agenda problem'.

progress with each of them it seems unlikely that we would be able to provide confident answers which were not dependent upon the broader social and ideological context of the health polity in question. I share these instincts and yet I think there are also good reasons to consider the issue in these most general of terms, or, more precisely, to also have the more general question in mind when focusing upon the more specific ones. My approach here is the one adopted throughout. We can and must ask and answer questions about obligations within specific institutional frameworks, but the answers we give must also take into account the social and policy contexts of these institutional frameworks. In this chapter I will begin by briefly reflecting on some of the different senses of responsibility and then I will return to consider in more depth the relationship between specific examples of questions about health responsibilities and the more overarching questions.

Senses of Responsibility

This is not the place to get bogged down with open-ended conceptual analysis but it is necessary to distinguish between different senses of responsibility; first between causal responsibility and ethical responsibility, and then between different senses of ethical responsibility (Dworkin, 1981). It is possible to distinguish between someone being implicated in a causal chain which results in ill-health and them having some ethical responsibility for that ill-health. If I prepare the meals in my household using a contaminated food product and cause serious food poisoning, I am certainly a key part of the causal chain that results in disease or death but, even though I may *feel* very guilty, I am not, by that fact alone, ethically responsible. To show that I was so responsible would entail either showing that I knew that the product was dangerous and that I nonetheless deliberately used it, or perhaps that I had failed to take the steps which might reasonably be expected to check its safety and that I had used it voluntarily. There are matters of degree relating both to what I might reasonably be expected to know about things and to the degree of control I have over what I do, but at least some minimum threshold of understanding and voluntariness is needed to turn causal responsibility into ethical responsibility. This food-poisoning example can also serve as a reminder that ethical responsibility is not of a single type, although the classifications we use here will depend upon our underlying ethical theory we can distinguish between different kinds of obligation and, in each case, between degrees of culpability. Have we, for instance, failed to do something we are ethically required to do? In a catering establishment there may be statutory requirements (which, let us imagine, there is a prima facie ethical obligation to follow) only to use certain food supply sources. If the owners freely choose not to comply with these requirements in exchange for a personal fleet of sports cars then they would find it difficult to deny ethical responsibility. By contrast, if a particularly perceptive employee has started to formulate a few doubts about the wholesomeness of the food-supply chain, but has as yet no evidence to back this up, and is under instructions to use the food as part of her job, her situation is very different indeed. We might say that 'high ethical standards' should entail some action on her part, e.g. that she 'makes a fuss' internally, that she reports the firm to the relevant authorities, that she resigns. But, depending upon the precise circumstances, we may not hold her to blame for the resulting food poisoning, or at most the level of blame ascribed to her would be relatively slight. In short we have a responsibility for those things which it would be wrong for us not to do, but we can also take some responsibility for those things where our actions could do some good or prevent some harm, even where we are not ethically required to act.

This example also illustrates the 'layers' of ethical questions about responsibility. For any agent we can ask, 'What ought she to do? What are the minimum and maximum ethical expectations others can reasonably have of her?' But we can also ask about the extent to which other people can ethically enforce or encourage the enactment of these responsibilities, and the rights and wrongs, benefits and harm, of different forms of enforcement or encouragement. It is widely understood that just because 'A ought to do X', it does not follow that it is ethically acceptable for B to make A do X. However, B may have various kinds of responsibility in relation to A doing X. (In the example the employer may have some responsibility for the conduct of the employee and vice versa). Various kinds of institutional and interpersonal rules and norms (including laws) can be used to articulate and underpin agents' ethical responsibilities and these rules and norms must themselves be subject to ethical scrutiny. This is also one of the themes of this chapter because debates about personal or professional responsibility for health are invariably accompanied by debates about systems of social sanctions or social accountability. Finally, in relation to the example, we can distinguish between asking 'Who is responsible for causing the food poisoning (including who is to blame)?' and 'Who is responsible for dealing with or responding to the food poisoning?' Questions about the past are different from questions about the present and the future. A specific person might hold the blame for creating a health need but many other people—passers by, ambulance staff, hospital staff, for example—may share a responsibility for meeting that need. Once the need so to speak 'comes into existence' their obligations are 'activated'.

Voluntary Health Risks and Healthcare Entitlement

A common focus within healthcare ethics for discussion of health-related obligations and entitlements is the question of allocating scarce resources to 'risk-takers' such as smokers or heavy drinkers. Within a healthcare system where there is pooling of resources, e.g. through state taxes or through a managed-care organization, should someone who smokes or drinks, and as a consequence of that behaviour, becomes unwell, be given the same priority as someone else with the same condition and the same other characteristics except for this behaviour? In this section I will briefly review some of the arguments rehearsed in these debates as a means of opening up the broader issues.[2] Even this comparatively narrow focus gives rise to a broad range of both theoretical and empirical complications. To begin with, the degree of voluntariness behind the risky behaviour will seem relevant to many people. In the extreme case where the behaviour was deemed to be entirely beyond the person's control then it could only be relevant to resource allocation if it makes a difference to the potential benefit of the intervention. It might be argued, for instance, that to give a scarce kidney to an alcoholic might be to relatively 'waste' its potential use, and this could be said without in any way attaching ethical responsibility to the individual for the alcoholism. But if we allow that these behaviours are to some degree voluntary (and the degree, of course, matters) then a number of other possibilities arise which are based upon acknowledging the risk-takers' responsibilities and not simply the effects of their habits on the utility of outcomes. In particular we can imagine trying to change these behaviours in various ways, by providing education, persuasion, or different forms of disincentives, or we could find means of 'penalizing' these behaviours if they continue. These provide us with some further possible reasons for giving lower priority to these risk-takers, such as: (a) preventive health measures depend upon sending clear signals about various risks and this is inconsistent with a climate of equal priority; (b) provided that understanding is sufficient and the conditions for a threshold of voluntariness are met then risk-takers have knowingly 'made themselves ill' and are therefore less ethically deserving than others who have 'looked after themselves'; (c) those who take voluntary health risks and understand what they are doing thereby knowingly raise their demand upon pooled resources, fairness requires that those who have chosen to avoid these risks (and thereby steward shared resources more carefully) should be given a higher priority all other things being equal. This then gives us four possible sets of reasons for giving smokers and heavy drinkers

---

[2] This section is particularly informed by the excellent discussions of these issues found in Wikler, 1987; Wilkinson, 1999; and Veatch, 2000.

lower priority in resource allocation: their ability to benefit from intervention; to support preventive healthcare, to penalize them for the choices they have made, and to 'restore'[3] fairness in the global distribution of burdens and benefits.

Each of these possible rationales for treating voluntary risk-takers differently gives rise to a set of puzzles in ethical theory and applied ethics, but they are all also bound up with a whole range of empirical uncertainties. Is our knowledge base about the determinants of health good enough to be able to disentangle the effects of certain behaviours, such that we could ascribe certain states of ill-health to certain behaviours (and could it be this good even in principle)? In practice would we know how to assess the relevant levels of voluntariness and understanding to ascribe ethical responsibility? Do we know enough about the overall healthcare costs associated with certain behaviours to determine when these entail creating more rather than less expenditure than would be expected in the absence of these behaviours? If one reason to 'discriminate' is the contribution it makes to preventive healthcare messages do we know enough about the effectiveness of these messages (and the relevant level of contribution made by healthcare access disincentives) to measure their effectiveness? None of these questions suggests, at least to me, the prospect of a simple affirmative answer. These are all extremely complex questions at or beyond the limits of social scientific understanding, and it is difficult to see how the levels of knowledge we do have about these things can form the basis for robust and fair policy-making. Nonetheless policies do have to be made in conditions of uncertainty and, in some cases, it is possible we may be able to develop a more secure foundation for our practical judgements. At the very least policy-makers ought to be expected to set out the working assumptions and hypotheses about these empirical questions which inform their decision-making.

Healthcare Entitlement in Context

I cannot treat either the theoretical or empirical questions summarized above in any depth, but I do want to discuss them a little further both to indicate their importance and to illustrate their relationship to the very general questions about health-related obligations and entitlements. First, the pivotal role of the empirical questions must be noted. Not only do the uncertainties in this area make it very difficult to ascribe causal responsibility for illness (smoking is more of an exception than a rule in this regard), but the elements of compulsion and/or the strong normative pressures surrounding

---

[3] Hence this is sometimes referred to as 'the restoration argument'.

some 'lifestyle choices' make it harder still to ascribe ethical responsibility with any confidence. Furthermore, even if we could make confident ascriptions of personal responsibility this simply moves us into empirical conundrums about the implications of these risk-taking behaviours for others. Assuming that we are only considering, for the time being, the self-harming aspects of these behaviours (and not their broader health effects) it is not clear how we should assess their 'cost' to others. A number of people have pointed out that smokers can be seen as less of a drain on common health resources than others because even though their average treatment costs per year may be higher than non-smokers their lifetime costs are lower because they live shorter lives on average. Thus any arguments that their healthcare entitlements should be reduced on the basis of 'fair expenditure' could be countered, and possibly reversed, given the comparative global 'cheapness' of smokers to health services.

The theoretical conundrums are equally complex. Each of the four kinds of reasons set out above deserve attention but they rest upon different possible ethical bases. Voluntary health risk-takers could be deterred from their behaviours for either *paternalistic* or *utilitarian* reasons, because better health is good for them personally, or because it is better (in various ways) for society; and/or they could be *blamed* and penalized for their recklessness and lack of prudence; and/or they could get *fair treatment* but this entails them being accorded a different priority than others (either because of their ability to benefit or their disproportionate demands on the system). As ever this kind of combination of possible reasons has to be treated with caution. On the one hand they can simply be fudged together into a general sense that the compound as a whole provides a justification, but if each of the reasons examined independently seems weak then we should not assume that they add up to something stronger. On the other hand it may sometimes be that there is an 'additive quality' to sets of reasons which mean that a relevant threshold of defensibility is reached when some of them are combined.

My prime interest here is in stressing that whatever we think about the merits of these different arguments their practical defensibility and their policy relevance depend upon us evaluating them against a background set of assumptions concerning health-related obligations and entitlements. That is, we can only evaluate these rationales against some more or less explicit model of health-related obligations and entitlements in general. (With, in turn, some conception of how this model can not only be defended in principle but also be achieved in practice.)

We might, for example, take the view that anyone who is ill and can receive some discernible benefit from healthcare treatment should have an equal chance of getting healthcare treatment regardless of any other factors, e.g. their personal history, their financial contribution to the health system, the degree of their ability to benefit. From this perspective none of the above arguments would have any purchase because none of the criteria reviewed in these arguments would have relevance. However, this, if we consider it for a few moments, is something of an extreme position and one that it would be an uphill task to justify. I will mention some of the obstacles quickly. First, very few people actually think that degree of benefit is irrelevant to the allocation of healthcare. Even if we think the extent of the potential to benefit is irrelevant within treatment groups we are are unlikely to think that the range and distribution of types of treatments are irrelevant and that everyone should have an equal chance of being treated no matter how 'trivial' or 'serious' the condition. In this way factors like 'severity of condition', and 'health outcomes' become central to macro-healthcare resource allocation. Second, the fairly widespread intuition that people should have, roughly speaking, equal access to healthcare (or equal access according to need, to accommodate the last point) normally rests upon a set of background assumptions about health-polity contingencies. Very often what is being articulated is the view that equal access is ethically important *as one of the rules of the health polity game.* Other rules of the game might be, for instance, that the individuals in question are fellow citizens, or more specifically that they have paid their taxes or insurance contributions. Where these other rules are broken the ethical force of the equal access judgement may weaken. Of course it is possible to argue that 'mere humanity' alone should be ethically sufficient but it is important to recognize in so doing that other ethical arguments (around citizenship conditions or fair terms of social cooperation) fall out of the picture. Third, for the reasons explored in Chapter 5, it is ethically odd to 'fixate' on equal access to healthcare, when what seems of more fundamental importance is equal access to 'health opportunity', where this involves consideration of the many determinants of health including, but transcending, healthcare treatment.

The point here is that there is no single, neutral, or clear 'background model' from which debates about healthcare entitlements can start. Equal access on the basis of equal need may, in certain climates, be a widely shared working assumption, but it is only one position which it is not unproblematic to defend or interpret. The same applies to any other possible working assumption. The point here is that the assessment of arguments that suggest that smokers should have 'reduced entitlements' depends on a consideration of not only (a) in what respects smokers are different, but also (b) what is a 'normal' entitlement and why? As we have seen this issue has quite immediate practical relevance. If one's entitlement is a function only of one's current state of health then being a smoker makes no difference; if it is partly a function of how much resource you are likely to use within a five-year budget period then smokers might have less immediate entitlement; and if it is a function of how much resource you are likely to use in a lifetime then smokers might have more entitlements in the short term. These kinds of considerations are, of course, reflected in private health insurance schemes where premiums tend to reflect certain known health risks. Within this 'pooling of risk' adjustments can be made to allow for the fact that not everyone is equally placed in relation to risk. In this way 'equal entitlements' may be broadly preserved in the meeting of need but adjustments made in the sharing of the costs. Of course this private insurance model, considered in isolation, means that overall healthcare entitlement is dependent upon ability to pay, and those who are both poorer and more at risk of ill-health are, in effect, doubly disadvantaged. By contrast in single payer 'welfare state' systems of healthcare funding the attempt is made to largely insulate health-care entitlement from personal circumstances.[4] Although there is always the possibility of exceptions under these systems the 'irrelevant' personal cirum-stances are normally taken to include 'lifestyle choices', such as smoking. Thus if we begin by asking questions about the implications for healthcare entitlements of voluntary health risks we are forced back onto considering the ethical bases of health polities considered as a whole.

That is why making progress with the kinds of arguments from which I began—the four possible reasons for treating smokers and heavy drinkers differently, and many other such arguments—depends upon us first and foremost interrogating our background model of health-related obligations and entitlements. We need to have at the front of our mind fundamental questions about the ways in which social and institutional frameworks determine health opportunities and experiences, the ways in which these social and institutional frameworks themselves construct health-related ob-ligations and entitlements, and the ethical defensibility of these arrange-ments. In relation to healthcare this means, for example, interrogating the ethical bases of different systems and mixes of funding and allocative au-thority. And this entails much more than a generalized debate about the advantages and disadvantages of 'the market' versus 'the state', or the respective roles of the private and public sector, or of more or less centralized or devolved models of priority setting. It means acknowledging that the broad-brush ethical arguments in favour of specific models require very close scrutiny and qualification, and that part of this scrutiny is a careful

---

[4] Although, of course, differences in access due to differences in social and economic capital are persistent whatever the system. This is a paradigm example of the need to differentiate between the 'myths and simplifications' built into discourses about health systems and the complex reality of embodied systems. The ideology of equity can easily subsist alongside multiple forms of discrimination and stigmatization. Obviously analogous 'myths and simplifications' exist in relation to such things as 'choice' and 'responsiveness' in market models.

examination of the real world *effects* of these social arrangements on health and other experiences.

One important set of questions here, as I have begun to suggest, are those about the social and institutional definition and boundaries of the healthcare system; i.e. what is supposed to be achieved by different models of framing and what is achieved in fact. So, for example, on the ideal type welfare-state model healthcare is supposedly removed from the vicissitudes of the rest of life, including the general competition for resources and goods. Similarly in the ideal-type market model healthcare is treated as a commodity like any other, and although some people will be better placed than others to consume healthcare, market mechanisms can be used to spread access to some extent. Advocates of these models, or more likely some much more subtle mix, are not necessarily claiming that they achieve everything that ought to be achieved by an ethically defensible healthcare system, but they may well claim that their favoured system is, given a particular context, the best system available. (The assumption this distinction rests upon is that social and institutional frameworks of healthcare are 'imperfect' even in principle, i.e. they cannot deliver at one and the same time all of the good things we would like them to deliver.)

Ethical appraisal requires the consideration of the organizing principles and effects of the whole healthcare system as well as the elements within it. And, from a public-health perspective, the healthcare system is only one aspect of the social and institutional 'production' of health. We should, therefore, consider the side effects of healthcare systems to include their contribution to broader expectations about the distribution of health responsibilities. Or to put it the other way round, and more positively, we can ask 'How ought the healthcare system be designed if it is viewed as one part of a global system of health-related obligations and entitlements?' Obviously, this chain of reasoning can and must go on further, health being only one part of a total polity which encompasses a range of other competing goods. And it would be incoherent to attempt to determine a defensible model of health-related obligations without regard to these other elements of the social and ethical context. This takes us back to the dauntingly large canvas with which I began the chapter.

Merely to illustrate some aspects of this larger canvas and its importance to healthcare ethics I will briefly return (here and at the close of the chapter) to the question of the best societal response to voluntary health risks. It should be evident that the best response to such things depends on both what we see as the relevant facts and the right ethical analysis of these facts. Two specific sets of questions are prominent: (i) in what respects do other people have 'a stake' in individuals' risk-taking behaviour, perhaps as 'causes' of it, or 'victims' of its consequences? and (ii) what, if any, ethical basis does this specific stakeholding give for 'interfering' in the lives of others, and what can be done to optimize the ethical acceptability of any potential interference? Out of the many possible answers to these questions come the different social and political theories through which specific issues, including issues in healthcare ethics, are analysed. In relation to the example under consideration we need to decide how far behaviour such as smoking or heavy drinking either are or ought to be treated as if they are purely private self-regarding choices or how far they are, or ought to be treated as if they are, other-regarding activities in the public realm. These questions are, all at once, empirical, philosophical, and political. That is to say they certainly have empirical components because they involve making some judgements about facts, causes, and effects, but the ways in which we conceptualize and analyse 'the facts' depends upon our philosophical frameworks (for example, should 'the fact' that individuals may be saddened because some people who are strangers to them self-harm count as relevant?). Finally, even if we take the view that, for example, massive paternalistic intervention with risk-taking behaviour was ethically defensible in principle we may still conclude, in specific sets of circumstances, that it is practically untenable, or is likely to do more harm than good. This is a practical political judgement which can be presented as falling either within or without ethics.

What is completely untenable is to treat certain positions here as if they are neutral, 'obvious', taken for granted starting points. The health promoter who takes it for granted that their efforts to prevent disease or promote health must be for the good, or the 'liberal individualist' who takes it for granted that his or her right is to be 'left alone' occupy the same ground. They are both equally happy to assert the primacy of some particular analytical framework without either subjecting that perspective to critique or recognizing that it may come into conflict with other equally important perspectives. In the real world these two perspectives inevitably conflict and neither can entirely trump the other one. Even advocates of the smallest role for the state or other public institutions will insist that individual action should be regulated for public 'health-protection' reasons. Even the most passionate public-health promoters will recognize that individuals need space if they are to have lives worth living. If we add to these commonplaces the fact that there are no clear boundaries between health protection and health promotion we have the beginnings of a sensible discussion.

A health polity represents a specific constellation of embodied answers to these balancing questions. The systems of health-related obligations and entitlements it defines reflect a view about the best means of reconciling and, where necessary, separating health as a public and private matter. The central problematic of this book is that health, however broadly or narrowly defined, and the whole set of health-related goods, has both an individual and a public face. Here health is just one example of the impossibility of a neat separation of the public and private spheres. Any settlement of the tension between health as a matter of public interest and health as a private interest is going to be a less than perfect, practical, and institutional one. We could, for example, attempt to 'police' the public domain so as to reduce as far as possible public-health risks whilst expecting individuals to take full responsibility for funding their own healthcare when they need it. This combination may seem to have many things to commend it, but such a sharp rupture gives rise to a significant number of anomalies both in principle and in practice. For example, certain kinds of treatment conspicuously 'fall down the middle' of this divide. (When someone is being treated for a sexually transmitted disease which side of the line are they on?) In practical terms patterns of motivation need to be considered, and motivational questions cannot be divorced from ethical ones. Why should an individual for whose healthcare costs the wider society has 'no responsibility', be inclined to cooperate with other-regarding health-protective measures and messages? Why, in explicitly ethical terms, should the scope of reciprocal political obligation and benefit extend through public health generally but stop at healthcare?

The 'Agenda Problem'

Before continuing I want to pull together the main issues discussed up to now through some brief methodological reflections. The issues I have in mind all relate to a familiar but fundamental problem in applied ethics which has been called, amongst other things the 'agenda problem' (Brock, 1987). This problem can be summarized in the form of the following question: 'Faced with a decision about what is the right or the best thing to do in situation S, what features of S should we take as a "given" and as thereby falling outside of the scope of consideration except as the context for the ethical deliberation?' This is not just a puzzle for applied ethicists, it is an extremely familiar problem in day-to-day practical ethics. For example, how far should I treat what I take to be the broadly well-founded demands of my professional code of ethics seriously in instances where I believe its requirements are misjudged? Should I treat it as a given which has at least some role, even if not a decisive one, in my ethical deliberations, or should I view it as a contingent feature of the landscape which I am seeking to change? And how far would my attempts to change the code in this regard, were I to make them, alter my obligations to follow the code in any case?

This particular example is directly related to the relationships between what I called 'internal and 'external' evaluation in Chapter 4. But because my overall focus is on the social context of healthcare ethics, the agenda problem is closely implicated in everything I am considering. The main way I have referred to it in this chapter is by saying that decisions about specific obligations and entitlements can only be made against background assumptions about wider patterns of obligations and entitlements.

Although the agenda problem is relevant to everyone its implications can look rather different when considered from the point of view of a practical agent as contrasted with an applied philosopher. Consider the case of a doctor who is expected to refuse treatments because of what she sees as a clearly unethical set of policies, e.g. a 'pro-choice' doctor in an anti-abortion climate and health system, or one working in a context where the most crass economic modelling of resource use has been adopted as a political imperative. What ought she to do? In one important sense she and an applied philosopher colleague are likely to agree about this. They may well agree that these policies ought not to be in place, that the world ought not to be the way that it is. They may also agree that the doctor, in concert with others, ought to take steps to challenge these policies. However, beyond this point the interests of the doctor and the applied philosopher are likely to diverge to some degree. There are few incentives for applied philosophers to dwell at greater length on the best ways of fulfilling one's professional role in these sorts of circumstances, whereas for the professionals themselves this is an inescapable and essentially important focus of concern. For this reason a 'fully' applied philosophy needs to consider the range of relevant agendas and vantage points: how the world might be better in various respects and how to act given that some of these things, at least, are not about to change. (In short critical ethics and conventional ethics cannot be neatly separated.)

Clearly the agenda problem is a major methodological consideration for applied ethics. It requires us to decide how much weight we should attach to the well-known joke response to being asked for directions: 'If I were you I wouldn't start from here.' The principles underlying the health polity could be different, the institutional frameworks and norms through which these principles are realized could be different, and if they were different the question to hand would not arise or would not arise in this form. This means that all ethical deliberation necessarily has both an imaginative and a strategic dimension. It involves working on the foreground and background together, and deciding when to concentrate on one more than the other. When, for example, should we act as if whatever the flaws of the prevailing health polity it is the least bad option practically available to us? All work in applied ethics has to find ways of managing the agenda problem although often this is done implicitly rather than explicitly.

In some work the agenda problem is addressed explicitly. For example, Erin and Harris's analysis of the duties of HIV-positive individuals sets these duties overtly in the context of a model of 'reciprocal obligations' (Erin and Harris, 1993) between individuals and the state. They argue, I suggest quite persuasively, that it makes little sense for us, as a community, to define the ethical obligations of such individuals to protect the health of the community unless, at the same time, we are ready to take steps to protect the interests of these individuals (privacy, employment rights, etc.) in return. They ask us to lift our gaze from the specific obligations of individual citizens so as to address the broader frameworks that make sense of such obligations.

Another example is Hardwig's much discussed argument (Hardwig, 2000) for a putative 'duty to die' which arises from an analogous shift in perspective. Can it make sense, he asks, for us to concentrate on an individual's entitlement to expensive medical treatment even if that means, in practice, that these costs will fall on a family whose quality of life will be ruined? We need to think, he suggests, in less individualistic terms and in a more family-centred way. Hardwig's critics (e.g. Humber and Almeder, 2000) serve equally well to illustrate the agenda problem. They do not resist the kind of shift in perspective he calls for, rather they question some of the contingencies from which he works, e.g. why assume that these costs have to be borne privately, and why limit the relevant constituency to the family? Why not rather consider individual entitlements in the context of population or global concerns? (This latter may, of course, serve to reinforce rather than undermine Hardwig's conclusion of a duty to die but I am leaving the substantive questions aside here.)

Here I need to acknowledge, and in so doing provide my final example, that the way in which I have constructed the concerns of this book 'screens out' the hugely important question of the individual and collective obligations of those of us in the affluent West to people in developing countries who face far more serious and pressing public-health problems. It is difficult to conceive of a more important issue for healthcare ethics than this one. (Perhaps, therefore, I should note in passing that I would want to use analogous and parallel arguments to those I have rehearsed in this chapter and the previous one, relating to a commitment to equal consideration and collective responsibility for health, to support a significant reorientation of concern, effort, and resources away from domestic-health agendas and towards international ones.)

The core methodological point I am stressing here is that an interest in identifying people's responsibilities, or in whether or not these responsibilities are being discharged, has to be combined with an interest in the contextual construction of these responsibilities, in how responsibilities are made and how they ought to be made.

Making Policy for Responsibility

For the rest of this chapter I want to consider the ethics of policy-making in this area. More specifically I want to look at the ways in which health and other public policies create networks of health-related obligations and entitlements, and consider the ethical defensibility of these processes. Once again I will focus on the distribution of responsibility for health, with emphasis on personal responsibility. But rather than starting from the question of 'A's responsibility for X', I will shift my attention to what I introduced earlier as B's responsibility in relation to A and X. How should policy-makers[5] make decisions about the construction of health responsibilities? When is it ethically acceptable, for example, to use incentives or disincentives to underpin what are deemed to be citizens' ethical responsibilities?

It is worth indicating, to begin with, that this is not a purely academic question. Policy mechanisms are routinely conceived of, and used, in these ways. Examples would include: witholding social benefits to parents who cannot demonstrate they have had their children vaccinated; fining 'absent fathers' who fail to contribute to the financial welfare of their children; setting targets for doctors relating to a measure of 'consumer satisfaction', or to rates achieved in screening programmes or treatment outcomes; and establishing and publishing 'league tables' of hospital performance. These kinds of policy mechanisms, and there are many, are designed to work in a variety of ways. They can engage people's motivation more or less crudely and so to speak through different 'channels'. At their most innocuous they can be presented as playing a broadly 'educational' role, for example, guidelines and perhaps certain targets might be seen as public reminders of reasonable expectations. Often, however, they have a simple 'carrot and stick' structure, the 'cost' of non-compliance with what is deemed one's public responsibility is spelled out as a deterrent or penalty. Between these two, however, there are other equally, or in some respects more, powerful forms of influence. Targets or league tables, for instance, can 'work' because they are linked to financial incentives and they can, at the same time, work because they appeal to people's sense of social identity, to institutional loyalties, to relative status, to feelings of pride or shame. More generally policy mechanisms can help to create and/or harness powerful sets of cultural expectations and social norms which exercise constraints upon, or

---

[5] To begin with I shall assume that 'policy-makers' represents an identifiable group of people who are charged with and properly authorized to determine policy. Of course in reality policy is made in different ways, by many different groups of people (including voters), often as part of an interactive policy process, and sometimes as part of a 'trade off' between vested interests or in ways which are not authorized or regulated by ideals. By contrast 'policy-makers' here refers to idealized agents or to idealized advisers to these agents. Of course the gap between the ideal and real accounts is ethically important in a number of respects.

become constitutive of, individual subjectivity and agency. (Here 'constraining' or 'being constitutive of' are a shorthand way of signalling the contribution of both sovereign and disciplinary forms of power, discussed in Chapter 3.)

It is a mistake to see the power of policy solely through the lens of either legal sanctions or economic controls because, although important, these things only represent one component of deliberation or motivation for individual or institutional agents. Policy-makers have themselves become increasingly aware of this fact, and often combine different types of power and influence to attempt to create the conditions and ends they are aiming at.

I would suggest that at some level, and in some respects, these kinds of policy mechanisms are clearly necessary and ethically acceptable. To deny this seems to be to imagine either that 'left alone' everyone would behave sufficiently responsibly, or that the harm or wrongs that would result from a laissez-faire system are somehow less significant than those which result from policies for 'responsibilization'.[6] There are not any, or at least I cannot see any, sharp ethical lines between the public regulation of professional standards on the one hand and the publication of targets or performance indicators for health professionals on the other. Equally it is not obvious to me that health professionals could be held to have public responsibilities with regard to health whilst other people were entirely exempt from these pressures. The question seems to boil down to specifics: what kinds of influence, on which people, and under which circumstances can be defended?

With regard to B doing Y to underpin A's doing X the following seem to be some relevant general considerations: 1. Does A have an obligation to do X?; 2. What kind of obligation is it; what will be the harm or wrongs caused by A failing to do X?; 3. How effective is Y likely to be?; 4. How coercive is Y, how much freedom of manoeuvre or scope for the imaginative exercise of autonomy does Y give A?; 5. How transparent are (a) the decision to do Y, (b) the process of Y?; 6. What are the 'side effects' of Y?; 7. How clear is B's authorization to do Y and what systems of accountability sustain B's decision-making authority? In effect the relevant considerations here are familiar from many other cases and circumstances.

This template of questions allows us to begin to make discriminations. I will illustrate this briefly through two contrasting examples. First, attaching penalities to doctors falling below certain minimal standards of care. Second, the government, in a welfare-state health system,[7] lowering healthcare en-

---

[6] This term is borrowed from Rose (1996) who uses it specifically to refer to the use of disciplinary power in liberal-democratic governance, but here I am using it more generically.

[7] Obviously the situation is different in a market model where market competition could allow some degree of competition for smokers' business on different terms. The question still arises, however, of how far the state should allow completely open competition if the result seems to marginalize some groups from equal access to healthcare.

titlements to smokers as a preventive healthcare measure (and possibly for some of the other reasons discussed above). This second example thus allows me to return to the case of voluntary health risks I have concentrated upon above. In the first case the doctors' obligations are fairly clear-cut. They have unambiguously 'signed up' to a social role and social institutions which require from them, as part of the deal, the provision of certain standards of care. Likewise the harm and wrongs that failing to meet this obligation entails are clear, immediate, and easily ascribable to these failings. Social penalties of various kinds are likely to work, and these penalities and their rationale are typically made perfectly transparent as part of the same 'professional regulation' process that creates the doctors' other entitlements and obligations. Finally, although these penalties work coercively they allow substantial room for autonomy beyond what are defined as the minimum standards. The second case looks completely different. The extent to which smokers have obligations to others to stop smoking for any reason is highly contestable. The extent to which they have an obligation to themselves, for the sake of their own health, even more so. It seems there must be many more effective ways of encouraging non-smoking than what will inevitably be, for most smokers, long-term 'threats' of lower priority healthcare. The problems of assessing the level of voluntariness of the smoking and the level of policy transparency to individuals (again bearing in mind the time period over which smoking causes ill-health) are manifold. Finally, there would have to be a good reason for singling out smokers for this attempt at social coercion. Not only is there no equivalent to the doctors 'volunteering' for special treatment but also the social effects of singling out smokers are troubling. It is not just that this may create or reinforce social prejudices against people who happen to smoke,[8] it is also that this effect would fall differentially on working-class people who tend (arguably for structural rather than entirely personal reasons) to smoke more.

Of course most cases of responsibilization will fall between these two examples. They will not be as easy to defend as basic professional regulation, but they will have more to recommend them than long-term threats to smokers of reduced healthcare access. What seems to me to emerge from the examples considered in this chapter is that we simply cannot make a tidy distinction between 'health-regarding' and 'non-health-regarding' actions, or

---

[8] Those people who are tempted to fall back on the restoration argument here as providing independent grounds for treating smokers differently because of their claim of an 'unfair share' of resources should read Wilkinson (1999). He successfully shows how this argument actually roots upon a stigmatizing or moralizing stance. Many other identifiable groups, e.g. firecrew and parents knowingly put themselves in a position of making higher demands on services but, because these things are deemed 'socially valuable', the restoration arguments are not applied. Hence it is the moralizing element not the restoration element that 'does the work' in the case for treating smokers differently.

between private and public action. And even if we could do this in principle then given the unstable and slippery nature of human action, the fact that actions can be conceptualized in multiple and often competing ways, we could not, in any case, neatly classify any action as of merely one type or another.

There is, I suggest, no such thing as wholly private or wholly public action. Each thing we do is both a step in our own biography and an enactment of our changing social identities and roles, and is implicated both causally and constitutively in the welfare of others, and this inevitably includes their health experiences. The lines of interaction may be relatively evident. If I happen to use a pension company which invests heavily in a major tobacco distributor, I am implicated in the fact that others smoke and thereby in their smoking-related illnesses (assuming that smoking is to some extent caused by the marketing of tobacco companies). Indeed, for these reasons it is possible that non-smokers are as causally responsible for smoking-related illness as smokers. But often these lines are much more diffuse and difficult to draw. Most generally speaking, given that health opportunites are partly a function of wider social structures, e.g. hierarchical patterns of access to education, employment, housing, etc., then each time my life choices are designed, consciously or unconsciously, to improve my place in these structures and thereby to reproduce the inequalities which they embody, then I am arguably contributing to the relatively poorer health opportunities of the less advantaged. (The fact that this is a diffuse connection and in certain respects contestable is not enough to eliminate its ethical relevance: to do the latter we would need to show precisely why it is irrelevant or misjudged.)

Policy-makers with an eye on the right distribution of health-related entitlements and obligation cannot, therefore, start by neatly separating the relevant 'health agents' from others, or the 'health system' from others.[9] There are practical reasons to make these distinctions in many instances. And making these distinctions may sometimes turn out to be wise for both practical and ethical reasons, but they are not 'natural' or neutral distinctions. So, to return to the questions about voluntary health risks and their relevance to healthcare entitlements, I want to say that actions which can be deemed to constitute voluntary health risks should be treated in exactly the same way, and examined through the same templates, as any other kinds of action. In each case the defensibility of responsibilization policies will depend upon many factors, and each case has to be seen in the context of the global distribution of health-related entitlements and obligations, and the social and

---

[9] And of course 'policy action' is as unstable and slippery as any other kind of action. In examining policy-making we need to be aware that policy-makers are 'doing' many other things than they say they are doing or that they are necessarily aware of doing.

institutional frameworks that define or underpin them. If, as I argued in the last chapter, public policy should be informed by a concern with protecting the health opportunities of the least advantaged then this entails a general obligation to the erosion or dismantling of the social arrangements that produce fewer good health opportunities for those who are already disadvantaged in other ways. But to the extent that such social reform is technically difficult, or that it involves widespread diminution of welfare in other respects, or other kinds of wrongs or unfairness, then this must have important implications for entitlements and obligations further 'downstream'. Otherwise unequal opportunities are simply further compounded at each level. Those people who have a 'better start' and better health prospects are more likely to continue to prosper, less likely to be able to need healthcare on average, and are more likely to be able to afford to buy their own healthcare.

It seems to me to be manifestly unjust to hold individuals responsible for the harm they may have done to their own health without also holding other people who are implicated in the causes of their illness equally responsible, at least in principle. Again, in principle, if we believe that we need educational measures in place for the former to ensure that there is the level of understanding necessary for ethical responsibility (or more coercive measures to 'enforce' ethical responsibility), then we should also be committed to educational or coercive measures for the latter. Finally, as I have just indicated, each of these measures has to be evaluated in the context of the others. In the case of smoking, for example, the first question to ask is 'How is each individual or institutional agent implicated in smoking-related illness?' Certainly the state, tobacco companies (their employees and other stakeholders), advertisers, citizens in general, and people who smoke can all be ascribed some responsibility because each of these agents could do things which make a difference here. Under these circumstances there may be some pragmatic policy reason to separate out smokers for certain interventions, but there is no clear basis for putting the whole ethical responsibility at their door. The same applies for all of the determinants of health and illness. We need to find a set of health-related policies which is based upon the recognition of this fact of diffused responsibility, and which does not differentially penalize those who may as often as not be the victims rather than the perpetrators of illness.

For healthcare ethics diffused responsibility means combining ethical analysis of policy contexts and institutions with work on individual professionals and citizens. We must examine and find ways of appraising the ethical bases and effects of the social and institutional arrangements which shape the production of health experiences and the distribution of health-related entitlements and obligations. Policy-making has to be evaluated through this lens, and the actions of individuals judged within this context. Each of these layers of appraisal is only relatively autonomous. Overall the judgements we make at each level determine the judgements we make at the others. In the next part of the book I will take a further look at these interdependencies by focusing on the changing roles and responsibilities of health professionals, and how these are constructed from, and interact with, both system-level and institutional norms.

Diffused responsibility also highlights another implication of recognizing health as a social good. It is not merely that policy has to be informed by a population-oriented approach to health. It is that we each of us have some kind of responsibility at the population level. Furthermore, if we accept the argument of the previous chapter, i.e. that the principle of equal consideration has to be applied to the social processes and institutions which underpin health, then each one of us arguably shares some responsibility for supporting systems and policies which underpin equal health opportunities.

PART 3

Institutions and Vocations

7

Professional Ethics in Context

To occupy a professional role is, of course, to occupy a socially constructed role. To acknowledge this is not to give way to wholesale social constructionism of the idealist variety. There is no need to suppose that social roles are not grounded in material facts or 'natural' human relationships, still less to suppose that these roles might be fashioned simply by the ways we choose to think or talk about things. Rather social things, including healthcare institutions and professional roles, are both 'real' and 'constructed', and the latter does not detract from the former, it just helps to explain it. (To borrow Searle's (1995) example, the substantiality and value of a banknote are not dissolved when we see that it is a product of a human institution.) This combination means that in order to understand occupational or professional roles, such as those of physician, surgeon, nurse, physiotherapist, pharmacist, health-service manager, and so on, we can look at them as if they were relatively fluid or relatively stable, and we can look at them—and this is not meant to be a sharp distinction—either from the 'outside' or the 'inside'.

The same professional roles change over time and space, and the historical and cultural processes which go to shape them are very complex (some of these will be mentioned below). But given a particular occasion and setting, and let us say a particular nursing role, we can ask both about the construction of the social identity in question, and about these nurses' own accounts of what they are about and their principles and purposes. In the first case we will need to consider such things as the evolving traditions of nursing; histories and patterns of recruitment, education and practice; the legal powers, restrictions, and definitions of nurses; the place of professional bodies and self-regulations including codes of conduct and informal norms; the expectations and working patterns specific to the setting in question; the relations of accountability and power and status hierarchies between different nurses, and between nurses and other occupational groups. In the second case we will need to try and make sense of, generally and specifically, what nurses hope to achieve through their work, the kinds of contribution they aim to make to the well-being of their patients, and what it is so to speak that they 'give' to their patients. Here we are, to some degree, dealing with nursing as a vocation, as one manifestation of a life lived well. Crudely speaking our sociological and historical impulses take us down the first path, our anthropological and philosophical ones take us down the second. At one end of the spectrum a sociologist might produce an account of a nursing role, for example, as a form of gendered oppression. At the other end of the spectrum a philosopher might seek to distil from the context-bound first-person accounts of nursing some 'ideal type' vision of the aims and character traits implicit in their conceptions of 'the good nurse', at least in the context in question.

But, as I have already indicated, there is no sharp distinction here. The internal vocational identity of nurses is not immune to historical or sociological explanations, nor are nurses or other health professionals, in a socially reflexive era, 'innocent' about the social and institutional contexts that shape their work. In this chapter I will focus on some of the tensions and interactions between what might be called the vocational and institutional identities of health professionals, between the ways in which they would like to think they act and the ways in which institutional regimes 'make' them act. For two reasons there is always likely to be some tension between vocational and institutional identities. First, social and occupational roles change over time and may change from the time someone considers entering an occupation to the time they become an established practitioner. Second, individuals will always have their own models and constructs of good practice, or at least their own emphases in interpreting these things, but social institutions need to find ways of coordinating the efforts of different actors in relation to some shared goals. As mentioned in the opening chapter one facet of the general increase in social reflexivity is the increasing prominence of health-service management and population-oriented goals as means of responding to the tensions caused both by historical change and by problems of social coordination. In the next two chapters I will use these respective examples of health-service management and public health/ health promotion to explore the changing nature of healthcare-professional ethics. In this chapter I will introduce these issues and will begin by making some general observations about the nature of healthcare professionalism.

Understanding and Evaluating Healthcare Professionalism

What it means to be a professional is something which is both highly contested and shifting. For example, commentators have distinguished between professionalization, professionality, and professionalism (e.g. Hoyle, 1980; Eraut, 1994). Professionalization is the social process that an occupational group has to go through to achieve certain forms of social status and a certain degree of power over an occupational domain. In this sense only certain groups might be properly called professional groups, archetypically doctors and lawyers, with other groups, such as nurses, achieving only a part or 'semi-professional' status. Professionality refers to the quality of doing one's job well, of adhering to the appropriate technical or ethical standards that meet the expectations generated by claiming to hold a certain occupational role. In this sense people in any occupational role can be more or less 'professional' in their practice. The notion of 'professionalism' can be seen as a compound of the other two notions. It is an ideological notion which, on most accounts, somehow marries together the social influence and the high standards. In summary this can be seen as a kind of contract between an occupational group and the broader society, and the ideology of professionalism can be presented in either an idealistic or a critical light. The former sees professional groups as being given social status and influence in return for them protecting the interests of the wider public within a particular occupational domain, by guaranteeing high standards of practice and delivering ideals such as altruism and service. The latter sees professionalism as a strategy of occupational exclusion and social control legitimated through a rhetoric of idealism.

Unsurprisingly this is an area where the insider and outsider accounts will tend to vary. On the whole doctors, for example, are unlikely to see themselves in as sceptical or cynical light as some of their critics. To get inside a professional role and to respond to its many demands normally requires a personal engagement with the goals and standards internal to the profession. Of course there will be many times when there are elements of scepticism or cynicism about these things, and times where individuals experience a significant gap between their personal agenda and their professional identity, but in the main there has to be a significant degree of congruence between personal identity and professional ideals. Here it is worth explicitly returning to what in Chapter 4 I labelled 'internal' and 'external' evaluation. Social institutions can be evaluated both in terms of internal processes and effects and in terms of external processes and effects. These two perspectives are, of course, only relatively independent of each other, but are worth distinguishing sometimes for analytical reasons. Consider marriage for example. We can consider its overall effects as a social institution; does it provide for social cohesion or social fragmentation, is it necessarily a patriarchal institution which fosters the exploitation of women, etc? Or we can consider the dynamics and quality of particular diverse marriages: do the partners value the marriage, if so why? What would they consider to be the purposes and ideals that frame these specific marriages, and how well do they live up to them? Here it is clear that the external and internal accounts cannot be completely insulated from one another but are also to some degree autonomous. In some cases an institution, perhaps certain armed services or prosecution services, for example, will be such that many individuals will refuse to be associated with them for reasons of conscience. (Some people will feel this way about almost any institution, certainly marriage, perhaps home ownership, etc.) But health-professional roles in themselves are not typically the focus of conscientious objection. Conscientious individuals will enter these roles, despite some possible reservations, with a view to making their own conduct within the role as acceptable as possible, and perhaps also with a view as to how they may be able to contribute to the general evolution of the role. That is, they will incorporate thinking about both internal and external evaluation into their approach to their own work.

Even from this brief excursion into ideas about professionalism it is obvious that there is no simple account to be given of the bases and status of professional ethics. As an aspect of healthcare professionalism, professional ethics is bound up both with professionality, with meeting ethical standards as one dimension of intrinsic quality, and also with professionalization, i.e. with preserving the roles, boundaries, and influence of professional groups. This point can be seen more clearly still if we reflect on the division of labour within healthcare. This is what I turn to next. My purpose in considering this topic is not to make an extended analysis of the healthcare professionalism but to begin to open up the relationship between the division of healthcare labour and professional ethics.

The Division of Ethical Labour

The work of healthcare is divided up in many ways. Obviously much relevant work is unpaid and undertaken by 'lay' individuals, and if health promotion is counted as health work then arguably everyone is involved or implicated. But even if we just consider paid work undertaken within clearly framed healthcare settings then the range of people involved and the complex principles of division are striking. In a large hospital there are many recognized but small healthcare specialisms such as clinical nutritionists or medical engineers, as well as people from large allied professions such as physiotherapists, occupational therapists, speech therapists, and so on, and then, of course, many well-established roles and specialisms within nursing and medicine, in addition to administrators and support staff of many kinds. The work is divided up within, between, and across these occupational groups in ways which are both traditional and at the same time under review and revision. The frequent debates about role boundaries and about the improvement of teamwork or 'interprofessionalism' are just some of the signs of the tension between tradition and change. Even if we leave the idea of professional power or vested interests out of consideration and try to imagine an 'ideal' division of labour we are faced with a dazzling puzzle. Some of the things we need to coordinate are: (a) different kinds of knowledge and skills, both clinical and non-clinical, and more or less specialized, (b) different kinds of functions, tasks, and ways of responding to and dealing with patients, (c) the balance between more generic caring, screening, or medicine and more specialist intervention (whether that means key-hole surgery or counselling), (d) role and task division between types of staff and within specific settings of intervention, and (e) lines of hierarchy and accountability that reflect kinds of expertise in general, experience and status within occupations, and the demands of multiprofessional settings and interventions. This is no mean feat and it seems that there must necessarily always be some problems of, and limitations in, patterns of coordination. But to see this as a problem of 'skill mix', as it is sometimes described, is only to see part of the picture, because the mix in question relates not only to skills, narrowly understood, but also to a division of ethical labour.

Different occupational roles occupy different positions in 'ethical space' in relation to both obligations and ideals. First, different occupational groups obviously have different powers, permissions, and requirements attached to them. And these are not simply socially sanctioned or legally defined but are grounded in role-specific sets of ethical obligations. Common restrictions about bodily touching or the breaching of the intimate realm are suspended, under certain conditions, in the case of some health professionals depending on the role and setting in question. And, to use an example metioned in Chapter 3, the powers that pharmacists have in relation to the handling and dissemination of medicines are specific to them. Second, different occupational roles, again suitably specified in relation to setting and function, embody different 'philosophies' of healthcare. Although it is important to avoid talking in generalities here, a surgeon performing a mastectomy represents a different face of healthcare from the specialist psychosocial oncology nurse who may work with the woman affected before and after the operation, even though the doctor and nurse may see each other as close colleagues. Roughly speaking we can say that a skill-mix choice about whether or not to have more or fewer of each of these roles, in this or similar examples, is a choice about the ideals of the health service in question. This point about the 'philosophical mix' of health services is often missed from discussions of healthcare policy or ethics, but is an everyday point of contention for health workers on the ground. Much of the tension surrounding staff planning and recruitment consists in debate about the nature of the healthcare that ought to be on offer.

One way to illustrate the socially embedded nature of healthcare ideals and the ways in which different professionals occupy different positions in ethical space[1] is to consider the contrasting positions—a contrast that is directly related to the substantive theme of this book—of health professionals in public-health roles as compared to those dealing with a specific patient list. (But I should stress that this is only one example of a general phenomenon.) Both the obligation-set and the governing ideals of a public-health doctor are clearly different from those of a doctor in a defined clinical practice who is interacting with specific individuals. These differences have been rehearsed before but can be summarized by saying that the former will generally be guided by population-based goals and impersonal conceptions of health whereas the latter has to respond to the particular claims of individuals and in so doing will prioritize a set of 'health goods' which are inevitably more person-centred.[2] Likewise the frameworks of evaluation which we would normally bring to these roles would be correspondingly different, whether we were interested in assessing health-related outputs or the ethics of professional practice. Clearly the balance of resources and relative influence a health system puts into these contrasting roles (or roles with comparable emphases) has a substantial influence in embodying and shaping the ideals of the system and the value field of healthcare-professional ethics.

Models of Healthcare Professionalism

Up to now I have placed most emphasis on noting what I have called the 'outside' perspective and the ways in which healthcare-occupational roles are socially constructed, defined, differentiated, and orchestrated. It is also essential to acknowledge the importance of the internal perspective, i.e. the sense that health professionals have of what they are for and about. To reiterate, I am not saying that these perspectives are not constructed from and sustained by social institutions of various kinds, quite the opposite, merely that they also deserve to be understood on their own terms. One way of approaching this is by considering some of the 'models' of professional–client relationships which have been discussed in the healthcare-ethics literature (e.g. Veatch, 1987; Callahan, 1998; Donovan, 2000). These models may be seen as more or less implicit or explicit. They form part of the taken-

---

[1] These positions I am suggesting are constructed in large part by the value fields in which professionals work and in particular the specific obligation-sets and ideal-sets which are constructed for different occupational groups. Although I am not discussing them here we can equally well imagine that there are characteristic occupational virtue-sets. Taken together we can imagine that professional ethics tends to start from socially defined sets of 'goals, obligations, and dispositions': this phrase can also be taken as a shorthand for the main axiological dimensions of ethics mentioned in Ch. 4.

[2] More precisely both parties (like all of us) have to balance these different perspectives together but the emphasis in the balance is very different.

for-granted norms of healthcare institutions and interactions, but they can also be self-consciously considered and adopted within projects of professional development.

The range of healthcare professional–patient relationships has been, at different times, modelled by comparison with just about every other possible kind of relationship. Doctors, for example, have been seen as being, in some respects, like parents, friends, partners, priests, engineers, shopkeepers, capitalists, police officers, criminals, etc. These different readings, as well as reflecting different practices, reflect different perceptions of the actual and potential caring and power relationships within healthcare, along with different extrinsic evaluations of healthcare institutions. But if we just focus on possible internal ideals, we can identify just a few major ideal types. We can see the health professional as, fundamentally, a 'contracted worker' of the patient, largely ready and willing to undertake the jobs the patient wishes carried out. We can see the health professional as the 'beneficient parent' of the patient, largely responsible for paternalistically determining what is in the health interests of the patient and what will be done. Or we can see the health professional as in a kind of 'partnership' with the patient, albeit perhaps an uneasy partnership in which the patient's wishes and the doctor's judgements are sometimes in conflict.

These crude models, once they are qualified by an accompanying professional ethic, will often merge into one another. There are ethical limits to what the contracted doctor will be prepared to do. And the most paternalistic doctor, who is by definition interested in the patient's well-being, will need to be sensitive to the values and wishes of the patient. Nonetheless these ideal types represent contrasting starting points and emphases, and will be more or less embedded in different healthcare settings. It is widely understood, for instance, that patients who pay their doctors directly for services are likely to expect a different kind of relationship with their doctors than those who do not. There are, of course, analogous debates within nursing and other health-professional roles. The caring role of the nurse can be seen in some ways as paternalistic (or parentalist, if we prefer), or in some ways as that of an agent of the patient or an extension of the patient's agency, or in some ways as a companion, friend, or partner for the patient. Again these models will merge together or combine in various ways (for example, the advocacy model sits somewhere between the latter two).

Taken at their most extreme these various professional–patient orientations give rise to very different mutual expectations and correspondingly different criteria for evaluation. Although it is only a very broad generalization the overarching story of twentieth-century healthcare in Western countries was that of a marked shift from more paternalistic orientations towards orientations which emphasize patient autonomy on either a contracted or partnership model. This story of gradual 'empowerment' was explored in Chapter 3 and represents a fundamental rethinking of the requirements of professional ethics.

At the beginning of the twenty-first century these issues are by no means settled, and the philosophical and practical contests between ideal type professional–patient relationship are as lively as ever. In particular the tensions between the influential discourses of evidence-based healthcare and person-centred healthcare have, if anything, only served to highlight the potential conflicts between professional paternalism and respect for patient autonomy, and to raise questions about the extent to which these are resolvable. In the remainder of the chapter I want to focus on some current dilemmas about the construction of professional roles and how this shapes the value field of, and thus the nature of, professional ethics. As I have indicated in this section this requires sensitivity to a broad agenda. I need to bear in mind the differences between the external and internal evaluation of roles and actions, the ways in which roles occupy different positions within ethical space and the problems of coordinating these roles, and also the shifting and competing models of professional–patient relationships. Because this is an extremely dense as well as a broad agenda I will focus on a concrete example.

A Pharmacist's Dilemma[3]

A terminally ill man is hospitalized and asks for some sleeping tablets.[4] He knows the type he wants, they are the ones which he uses all the time at home. The hospital pharmacist (Steve) makes available a generic equivalent, which is pharmacologically identical but differently 'branded' and packaged, because the preferred tablets are not in the hospital formulary. The patient is distressed as a result and Steve's and other staff's attempts to reassure him that the prescribed drugs are 'the same thing' are unsuccessful. On hearing this Steve faces a choice; should he try to obtain the preferred drugs or should he decide that he is already doing all that he can in the situation? Obviously, in reality, the way in which we would analyse and evaluate the pharmacist's decisions and actions would depend upon knowing more about the circumstances of the case. In this discussion, in order to explore some hypothetical issues, I will just focus upon a few possible elements of these circumstances at a time, and shift both the story and my gaze as I go along.

---

[3] This is based on a real case (see Barber, 1991) although many aspects of the way it is presented here, and the surrounding speculations are completely fictionalized. My thanks to Nick Barber for permission to use it.

[4] This example assumes that the patient is not directly buying the treatment in question, under these conditions many, but not all, of the considerations which follow would be altered.

Let us suppose that Steve has for some reason found a way of conceptualizing 'what is at stake' in fairly clear terms. In his own mind he is clear that the patient's clinical needs, with respect to these tablets, are fully met by what has been prescribed but that the patient, equally clearly, has unmet wants, albeit in some sense unreasonable ones, and unmet wants which seem to be undermining his peace of mind at the end of his life. In these circumstances what would we make of Steve feeling sympathetic to the man, and feeling that he perhaps ought to do more, but deciding not to do so (more or less self-consciously) because: (a) it is a very busy day and there are many other competing demands on his time that need attention and/or (b) the chief hospital pharmacist tells him that the hospital policies rule out adding this 'unnecessary drug' to the formulary and/or (c) he examines his relevant professional code of ethics and good practice, and satisfies himself that his conduct has definitely met the standards set out in them? Even if we believe that the preferred drug ought to have been obtained and prescribed it seems to me that we have to view all of these reasons as relevant to our ethical appraisal of Steve's decision.

Issues of practicability and institutional and professional norms are, I am asserting, constitutive of professional ethics. This is not, at all, to say that what ought to be done is defined by 'custom and practice' or prevailing norms. I am happy to go along with all those ethicists who believe that serious ethics begins by questioning these things. However, it is to say that there are limits to the extent to which, and the range of circumstances under which, an individual health professional can ethically defend active departures from normal expectations. Of course Steve may have a separate obligation, as discussed in the last chapter, to challenge the hospital policies or to seek a revision of his profession's codes of practice, but he also has at least a prima facie obligation to fall in line with these things in the meantime. This latter obligation may well be overridden by more important considerations on occasions, but not anything can count as an exception. Otherwise the coordinated systems of healthcare and the mutual expectations that these embody and sustain would collapse.

As I have argued earlier in the book this point has very substantial implications for healthcare ethics. It means that healthcare ethicists cannot simply focus upon what an ideal actor ought to do under ideal circumstances, nor even upon how the circumstances ought to be reformed in order to support ethical action, but also need to grapple with what ought to be done (what is ideal, what is acceptable, what is blameworthy, etc.) for specific individuals under existing 'real-world' circumstances. And in turn, I suggest, this means that at least some healthcare ethicists, as is increasingly happening, need to be prepared to engage closely with the lived experiences and institutional realities of healthcare. One methodological feature of this closer engagement is, as I am trying to illustrate here, an awareness of the fact that the yardsticks for ethical evaluation are partly, and necessarily, a function of the specific role in question and the ways in which that role is socially defined.

Let us now suppose that Steve is himself the chief hospital pharmacist, and has a major role in determining the policies concerning the hospital formulary. Let us imagine that he is not only in a good position to press for treating this patient as an exception, but more generally is in a position to help revise the policies so that they are more flexible with respect to cases of this sort. His dilemma now takes this form: on the one hand he sees that the policies are perhaps too narrowly defined around the safety, effectiveness, and pharmacological properties of medicines. They do not sufficiently take into account other considerations such as the drug preferences of patients, which might sometimes be relevant to the well-being of patients. The costs to the hospital of obtaining and supplying this patient with his preferred tablets would be minuscule in relation to the hospital drugs budget (after all they are only sleeping tablets and he is dying). On the other hand he has a strong sense of the need to define policies so as to steward resources for the hospital population as a whole, and he believes that the main criteria by which this is done must be clinical, and that 'unreasonable' patient preferences can have at most only a marginal role. Furthermore he sees that the hospital procedures on which he and his staff rely mean that he cannot simply purchase an extra drug without having to invest time in extending the computerized purchasing, storage, and dispensing systems, and this means a much larger investment of time, effort, and money than the idea of 'buying a few sleeping tablets' suggests. Finally, he reasons, that although the 'costs' may seem worth absorbing in this particular case, if the policy was made more widely responsive to patient preferences the overall costs would be unsustainable. On balance he decides not only not to supply the preferred tablets but also not to significantly revise the underlying policies. How should we assess these conclusions?

As with the first scenario, we must consider the immediate constraints and normative pressures under which he is working. It may be that Steve's budget is already overspent and he is in the process of trying to find ways of restricting the formulary rather than extending it. It could be that the relevant hospital manager points out that she would be positively hostile to any increased flexibility in hospital purchasing at that time. Again, we can to some extent leave on one side the question of whether these constraints and pressures are defensible. It is Steve's job, as chief hospital pharmacist, to do the best job he can in the situation in which he finds himself, and that means there are limits to how far he can justifiably ignore or override the constraints presented to him. Of course, once again, there are very different limits to how far he can separately criticize them or seek to change them. We can now turn to this yet broader perspective and ask what principles ought to inform the setting up of a formulary in this kind of situation, in particular how far should patient preferences be accommodated, and what kinds of institutional constraints on principles of purchasing can be defended?

The main answer to these broader questions, I suggest, flows fairly obviously from the discussions in the last section of the chapter. Namely, it all depends on what models of professionalism and healthcare organization we have in mind. On some models of healthcare professional–client relationship the expectation is that the professional will be highly responsive to the client's perspectives and preferences, on others the professional will be more paternalistic, and hesitate less when discounting what they see as irrelevant or unreasonable patient agendas. Also, as indicated above, these models are not simply 'chosen' by individual professionals but are, to varying degrees embedded in the way certain roles are socially and institutionally defined. For example, in this case the other, less powerful, pharmacy staff have very little choice with regards to the central issue in question. These processes of social and institutional design have to respond to the interests of a whole population of potential patients, and thus have to balance together population and individual goods, whether these be the interests of all payers in an insurance scheme or of a local population within a single payer, state-organized, system.

The construction of a hospital formulary and associated issues in professional ethics, therefore, have to be seen in the light of many factors. I have used this example to illustrate, once more, the need for multilevel analysis in healthcare ethics. The analysis of the ethical dilemma facing Steve, and equivalent dilemmas, depend upon a parallel analysis of the political philosophies and the models of professionalism embedded in healthcare systems and settings. One important feature of different models of professionalism, highlighted by this example, are the competing directions and balances in professional accountability. Is Steve mainly accountable to a specific patient, to a group of patients, to an institution or manager, to his professional body, or to the wider society more or less democratically operationalized?

The example considered in this section also illustrates the relevance of 'structuration theory', as introduced in Chapter 1, to healthcare ethics, and its close relationship with the agenda problem discussed in the last chapter. The option-set which faces agents is a function of the structures and cultures in which they work and which more or less closely define their roles. It is normally neither practically possible, nor sometimes even a meaningful option, for them to step outside this framework. However, these social frameworks of action are not merely 'givens', they are themselves a product of collective agency and are, considered over time, reproduced or changed by agency. Finally, it must be stressed that not any kind of change is practicable, and hence that there is a limit to how far alternative 'hypothetical' realities can be used to justify immediate actions. As I set out in the general discussion of responsibilities in Chapter 6, when we think about professional ethics we need to think both about the ethics of 'role-holders' and about 'policy ethics', i.e. the ways in which agency of various kinds, and the processes in which agents are bound up, shape, and ought to shape, the construction of roles.

Value Allocation and Professional Dilemmas

What this multilevel analysis highlights, I suggest, is that much that is 'transacted' or 'performed' in the domain of professional ethics is not deliberated about or 'chosen', indeed it is very often not even brought to the consciousness of the professionals involved. In relation to any specific scenario there is much that can, and in large measure must, remain unexamined. The value field of health-related action is more or less given and the positions in ethical space occupied by the participants more or less laid down. In addition there are many other policy-related or institutional norms and constraints which, in one way or another, influence the range of action and the broad 'costs and benefits' of options within the defined option-set. Within these frameworks there is, of course, much that particular actors might do, but, and this is the crucial point, there is much that they do, so to speak, simply by and through being embedded in these frameworks.

Here I will borrow the notion of 'value allocation' from political science (see Easton, 1953) to characterize this phenomenon. If what we are interested in is 'Who gets what "good things", and where, when, how, and why these good things are allocated' (to paraphrase David Easton's famous account of politics) then we need to see questions about ethical action in the context of value allocation more generally. As I have just noted values are allocated in healthcare relationships both through the practice of professional ethics and through the ways in which the option-set of professional ethics is constructed. We can examine this by reference to a routine and superficially trivial example, an example which also illuminates something about the division of ethical labour in healthcare and the way it is constructed.

Jenny visits the hospital as an out-patient every three months for a series of tests designed to monitor and plan the ongoing treatment of a chronic illness.[5] When the monitoring regime began 15 years ago Jenny typically

---

[5] I am not going to specify details here because I want to make some broad-brush points about the structuring of professional ethics; furthermore I am going to assume all kinds of substantive points about possible policy changes for the sake of making these points. Of course real-world cases will vary greatly and will often not correspond with the substantive points I happen to make in the example.

only dealt with two people on her visits, a member of the reception staff and her doctor who would spend 15 or 20 minutes with Jenny undertaking 2 or 3 tests and discussing the continuing management of the condition. These days Jenny sometimes sees as many as six people, including nurses and technicians who undertake much of the monitoring regime and typically sees the consultant (or a deputy) for no more than 5 minutes. These changes have come about for a variety of well-known reasons, including the introduction of new tests and equipment, the need to organize out-patient clinics in a cost-effective way and, in particular, the decision to protect and circumscribe the role of the hospital consultant as a 'scarce resource' given mounting pressures on costs. Let us suppose for the sake of argument that all of the changes are underpinned by carefully considered technical and 'workforce planning' considerations. For Jenny these changes have affected her experience of the hospital visits—this much is obvious. What is a little less obvious is the ways in which the changes have reconfigured the performance of professional ethics.

From Jenny's point of view her hospital visits now feel less satisfactory, less personalized, more fragmentary, more like she is being 'processed'. From a pure disease-management perspective we might assume that the new system is as good (or better) than ever, but from the perspective of 'illness management', at least as seen through Jenny's eyes, the system has declined. Jenny feels the need for her occasional contact with the hospital to provide her with 'a conversation' about her illness and its management. Her daily experience of her symptoms and of treatments and their side effects provides her with material that she would like to share and 'review' with those responsible for her care. In addition she feels the need to explore the data yielded by the various tests, their possible implications for her treatment and prognosis, and their relationships with her day-to-day experiences. Jenny feels that the older system served these illness management needs better.

After consideration of this case we might come to the conclusion that the quality of healthcare provision has been adversely affected by the changes described. As I have set it out the provision has been redesigned to serve particular instrumental objectives. And as a 'side effect' extra healthcare professionals have been brought into the scene and some of the room for responsiveness to patient agendas may have been displaced. But judgements about quality are not necessarily or directly judgements about ethics. Why would I want to say that these changes alter the performance of professional ethics?

We can assume that professional ethics is unaltered in many important respects, for example, that the professionals involved are as honest and respectful as ever, and as motivated by and concerned about ethical conduct and their patient's welfare. I am not, at least not in relation to this example, interested in a thesis about 'the erosion of professional integrity'. Rather I am interested in how the 'hospital encounter' has been reoriented in this, comparatively trivial, kind of example. Whilst the conduct of all those involved may meet the best ethical standards the framework for conduct has changed. The changes described have reshaped the ethical space of the out-patient clinic. The staff who have been there for many years now work under a different set of constraints, face different expectations, develop new sets of habits, and are accountable in new ways. One of these differences is their relationship to colleagues in novel occupational and professional roles (new positions in the ethical space of the clinic). This is, in short, an example of the way that policy and organizational contexts shape the goals, obligations, and dispositions of healthcare workers.

The performance of professional ethics depends both upon how 'ethical positions' are constructed and how they are enacted; or more crudely on both context and conduct. Of course to say that professional ethics is changed is not to make an evaluative judgement. To evaluate these changes we would need to know more. For example, are the nurses and technical staff encountered in a position: (a) to discuss test data, and their potential implications with patients or (b) to have conversations with patients about their experiences and concerns? In short we need to know how the goals, obligations, and dispositions of these staff are institutionally shaped and practically realized. For example, if these members of staff are not authorized to discuss test results with patients they will have to wrestle with how far their caring response to patients can be made compatible with having access to knowledge that they cannot share with patients. And if they are authorized in this regard they will have to consider how far they are in a position to 'handle' what may be the substantial psychological consequences of test information on patients, or perhaps how they can best ensure that their responses are broadly in harmony with other members of the healthcare team. But, whatever the possibilities and problems here, what is clear is that the ethical judgements that these professionals come to think about, the ethical dilemmas that become prominent in their considerations and discussions will, to a large extent, be a product of the way their roles and relationships are socially defined. Thus professional dilemmas can be seen as a surface feature of the wider processes of value allocation.

Conclusion

As I said at the start of the chapter the subject of professional ethics requires us to consider both 'inside' and 'outside' perspectives. We have to take seriously first-person points of view (including vocational identities) as well as seeing questions from more 'distant' or 'detached' points of view, including not only the institutional and system-level construction of identities but also the perspectives of analytical and critical ethics. In the chapter as a whole I have tried to indicate something about how these things fit together. In this final section I will attempt to summarize this approach to analysing professional ethics, an approach I will follow in the two chapters following this one.

The changes that have and are taking place in the value field of healthcare reshape the context and the nature of professional ethics. They directly affect what I have called 'value allocation' and, by creating new ethical spaces and new positions in ethical space, they also reconfigure professional ethics. From the 'outside' we can say, to summarize, that new clusters of goals, obligations, and dispositions are fostered (whereas other clusters are relatively speaking displaced) alongside new sets of institutional norms and constraints. From the 'inside' these changes may create dissonance, for example, between vocational biographies and reworked institutional roles, but may just as likely create new forms of 'commonsense', new taken-for-granted frameworks for deliberation and decision-making. Furthermore, as I have tried to make clear, it is not enough to treat these first-person perspectives as merely relevant to 'customary' or 'conventional' ethics (Peters, 1981; Oakeshott,1962) as opposed to the 'real' ethics that might be discerned through more philosophically rigorous reasoning. At the very least individual professionals have an obligation to treat the social frameworks which define their roles with great seriousness (and this is to say something more than that they are necessarily absorbed into these frameworks), i.e. professional ethics has to keep its feet on the ground of customary ethics. But, from the outside, it is possible to see that changes in customary ethics produce changes in what so to speak comes to the 'surface' of ethics, that is in what kinds of dilemmas are crystallized and made visible, and at the same time in what ethical hazards are obscured. One of the functions of critical healthcare ethics is to investigate the relationships between the more and the less visible features of the ethical landscape. Along with others I have relied on a particularly notable example here, namely the relationship between the rise of 'priority setting' cultures (visible dilemmas) and the consequent worries about the quality of (and specifically trust in) professional–patient relationships (ethical hazards). But this is, as I say, just a notable example of the relationship between healthcare change and the reconfiguration of professional ethics.

It would not be sensible to attempt to describe all of the relevant changes here. There are so many, they are complex, they do not form a coherent set, they vary from health polity to health polity and, finally, any descriptions of them will be hotly contested. But some of the main dimensions of change are familiar from other parts of the book. They include the opening up of the 'philosophical skill-mix' of healthcare and the growing prominence of public-health perspectives such as those, for example, about health promotion and prevention—those things that make up the widening and deepening of the diffused health agenda. Overlapping with these broad shifts are the many reforming discourses which serve both to express, but also in some cases to check, these diffusing tendencies, not just discourses around holism or person-centredness, for instance, but also the discourses of priority setting, of governance, of evidence-based healthcare, etc. And, alongside these discursive shifts are the multiple structural and organizational reforms which embody and 'contain' healthcare policies and practices, securing cost-containment but also delivering new forms of accountability to 'consumers' and funders, with larger roles for managers and markets. Each of these things constructs the value field of healthcare and thereby reshapes the ethical spaces in which health professionals work. The example about Jenny, above, picks up on just one facet of these manifold changes, the move, at least in certain parts of modern healthcare systems towards 'routinization.'[6] To the extent that it has taken place in certain sectors routinization represents two potentially important trends in professional ethics. First, a tendency for professionals to act as institutional rather than individual agents, as cogs in the institutional machine. Secondly, a tendency for 'technical rationalities' to displace 'substantive rationalities' (Yeatman, 1987), i.e. for decision-making to be led by a narrow outcome-oriented, instrumental, measurement-led kind of reasoning, rather than by a 'thicker', more contestable, but also more reflective engagement with the intrinsic goods of healthcare.[7] The two sets of tensions, between individual and institutional agency and between technical and substantive rationalities, are evident in the longer case study in this chapter about Steve, the pharmacist. They are also explored in more depth in the following two chapters which consider professional ethics in relation to two of the broad changes listed above, the growth of healthcare management and the discourses of health promotion.

---

[6] The extent to which routinization involves deprofessionalization (or even 'proletarianization') is much debated; as is the question of the extent to which it involves a fundamental shift of power from doctors to managers or others, but the existence of some trends in these directions seems undeniable. Eliot Freidson (2001), for example, has contested generalizations of this kind arguing that doctors, *considered as a whole group*, have found means of retaining their professional power, although they have done so by the development of new forms of routinization and stratification *within* the medical profession.

[7] Compare Macintyre's (1985) conception of 'internal goods', i.e. the goods that are internal to, bound up with, and only realizable through our practices. You can only experience, express, and communicate the goods internal to music (or healthcare) through the practices of music (or healthcare); and these need to be contrasted with success in relation to external indicators.

8

Managing Healthcare: Making or Breaking Healthcare Goods?

Health-service management is an unquestionably important field in its own right. As I mentioned in the last chapter coordinating activities across a complex division of healthcare labour is a necessary and challenging task. The more the quality of healthcare is researched and theorized the more the importance of effective teamwork within and across professions is recognized; and this teamwork depends upon effective management approaches and systems. What is more, the skilful management of non-human resources, budgets, equipment, drugs, etc., is equally essential. Indeed the stewardship of scarce resources is often presented as the central concern of health-service managers. This issue has risen up national agendas as part of the 'crisis' in healthcare costs associated with changing demographics, new technologies, and increasing demand. Whether this is seen as part of the control of public-sector finances or as a tightening up of shared insurance expenditures (such as in managed care models) health professionals are increasingly subject to management constraints on costs.

In what follows I will look more closely at some of the ways in which forms of management shape professional roles and professional ethics. But I also want to use this chapter to consider the ways in which management itself represents an increasingly important form of healthcare agency. Management is a key contributor to the reconfiguration of the value field of healthcare, although, as I hope to show, it can also perform crucial legitimating functions that tend to mask its considerable effects on both political and ethical agendas. This chapter, therefore, concentrates largely upon the importance of management (and 'managerialism') for the value field of healthcare, and for health-professional ethics in particular. It is not expressly about substantive or specific issues in 'management ethics' although I will touch upon some of these in passing. Rather it is about investigating the importance of what is represented by 'management ethics' in general, i.e. a concern with more general, impersonal, or population-oriented imperatives or obligations than those normally associated with individual health professionals.

Health-service management is one instance of the responsibilization mechanisms discussed in Chapter 6. Management pressures serve both to define
and underpin what are deemed to be the appropriate lines of accountability,
priorities, and patterns of obligations of healthcare institutions and of health
professionals. They help, for example, to determine what it is acceptable or
unacceptable for a professional to do within a particular context and, as the
previous chapter showed, what models of professional–client relationship are
enabled or emphasized within that context. They provide a clear instance of
the social construction of professional roles. For all of these reasons the rise
in health-service management has been very controversial. Health professionals, particularly doctors, who have tended to stress a relatively autonomous conception of professionalism, valued because of its intrinsic qualities,
have seen managerial influences as a threat to their professional identity,
influence, and to the basis of professional–client relationships.

The interactions between management, health policy, and healthcare professionalism are many and varied, and can be analysed from a range of
perspectives. I can only indicate a few key issues here. One way of opening
up this area is to note that management has to combine a concern with both
external and internal evaluation, and with both institutional and vocational
identities. The management perspective has to be sensitive to system needs
and to the role of healthcare institutions within systems, but it also has to be
sensitive to the perspectives of professionals and patients who are focusing
on the intrinsic goods of healthcare. I say 'the management perspective'
rather than 'the perspective of managers' because it is important to distinguish between management as a process and management as a specific
occupational role. Although some people are employed as managers full
time, there are many others, including doctors, nurses, and other professionals, who have some managerial function. Indeed, as I will discuss further
below, it is plausible to assert that fewer and fewer people fall outside the
form of social reflexivity and collective surveillance represented by management. Management, understood most generally, is simply one kind of collective agency aimed at the coordination of purposes and procedures. In
health-service contexts this means, amongst other things, looking for ways
to marry the 'policy effectiveness' of institutions with the vocations of
individuals.

Managerialism and its Ethical Implications

I am using the expression 'policy effectiveness' to highlight the fact that the
models and measures of effectiveness that institutions (and institutional
units) are subject to are largely a product of the healthcare-policy context.

Although there is some room for institutions to determine their own goals and priorities, and thereby to shape their own notions of 'success', both the regulatory and the competitive/comparative arenas in which healthcare institutions operate mean that much of the evaluative lens through which institutions see themselves arises from the wider policy framework. Indeed, it would be no great exaggeration to say that management is the name for the process by which the broader structural and cultural changes that take place in health polities and systems are mediated into, and made real in, the lives of institutions.[1] All healthcare institutions thus need to be 'policy effective' in two senses—they must be effective in responding to the changing demands of the policy context, and in particular they must have regard to the measures of performance that are made salient by the prevailing policy context.

Managers and management mechanisms, whether narrowly or broadly understood, therefore, have a key role in realizing policy change at 'ground level'. If reforming discourses, such as the ones around evidence-based healthcare, are to have a substantial effect on day-to-day healthcare practices they have to be operationalized or 'managed'. But to put things like this is potentially misleading. It might suggest that management is largely a kind of neutral toolkit that is used to translate policies into practice. It is better, I would suggest, to see the growth in scale and influence of health-service management as itself a central component of recent trends in healthcare policy, and as a component that in many ways embodies, and helps 'hold together', major changes in the values and ethics of healthcare. Clarke and Newman (1997) use the expression 'managerialism' to capture the currently prevalent idea that what is needed in welfare services is 'more and better management', and the way this idea has grown as an ideology. Although their analysis relates primarily to public-sector restructuring in the UK, and hence to policy change in what were, formerly, welfare states, its relevance, as I will illustrate below, is much broader.

The rise in social reflexivity and the diffusion of the health agenda, reviewed in Chapter 1, both require and enable new modes of social coordination. If systems and institutions are to be effective they need to 'contain' the potential diversification, or unravelling, of agendas associated with more awareness of the social dimensions of health and the accompanying processes of diffusion. In simple terms institutions cannot address all aspects of 'breadth' and 'depth' at once. Faced, as they are, with a proliferation of concerns with prima facie relevance they have to find methods of focusing down. This focusing encompasses more than the issue of priority setting or

---

[1] This is not to imply that management cannot play a role in resisting policy changes: both the tensions between policies and the conflicts between embracing and resisting policy change are 'worked through / fought out' at every level of the system.

cost-containment narrowly understood. It also relates to the degree of responsiveness of institutional agendas to broader 'philosophical' changes in healthcare such as those about responding to determinants of health or prevention, treating patient subjectivities seriously, lay involvement in decision-making, tackling inequalities, etc. And management is itself one expression of social reflexivity: it represents the official self-consciousness of institutions, a particular kind of self-consciousness which is in part facilitated by the growth in information systems and by ever more pervasive practices of review, evaluation, and audit.

The growth of managerialism is one facet of the rise in checks and balances which have been set against health-professional authority and autonomy. In the context of the welfare state model[2] this has involved a relative decrease in the combined power of health-service bureaucrats and health professionals and a comparable increase in the power of managers. Models of management, typically mixed in with models of market-thinking, have been borrowed from private and commercial sectors so as to meet the real and perceived problems of welfarism, e.g. problems of responsiveness and choice, and, most prominently, to underpin system and institutional 'efficiency' and 'value for money'. Thus although the diagnosis of the maladies of the welfare state and more market-based healthcare systems may differ, a broadly similar remedy has been put in place in all developed health systems, namely a tightening up of managerial control over potential 'waywardness' produced either by individual professionals or by 'unmanaged' system-effects.

In the remainder of this section I will try to spell out the implications of managerialist ideology, and related forms of institutional self-consciousness, for health policy and for healthcare ethics. In a nutshell, I suggest, these implications stem from the need for management to tell certain kinds of coherent stories about institutions: stories which are not only relatively simple but are, whenever possible, relatively simple stories of success. I hope I have said enough already to indicate that health-service management performs necessary and valuable functions, and that good healthcare depends upon good management, but I am now placing the emphasis on a more critical reading of two overlapping tendencies within managerialism (i) the imperative to measure, and to achieve success in, institutional performance and (ii) the associated technicist–instrumentalist nexus of languages and practices which displaces or transfigures ethical and political judgements into judgements about 'effectiveness' or similar notions.

---

[2] Clarke and Newman (1997) develop the analysis which I am drawing upon in this section as part of an account of a transition between the welfare state and what they label 'the managerial state'.

Performance measures. Health-service managers are subject to, and subject others to, multifarious measures of individual or institutional 'performance'. The ability to steer institutional strategy and control professional behaviour depends upon managers being held accountable both for budgets and for meeting relevant performance measures. In this way management is able to translate institutional priorities into the practices that allow their institutions to survive or succeed in the comparative/competitive arenas of the health polity, whether these represent 'indirect' market comparison such as published league tables of performance indicators, or more direct measures of relevant market share.

The displacement of value-disputes. One of the major effects of a managerialist mode of coordination is the relative displacement of, or effacement of, the countless value-disputes that are embedded in health policy and healthcare. This comes about because of two interacting factors. First, there is an inevitable component of reductionism both in the performance measures which inform external and internal policies, and in the technicist–instrumentalist kinds of reasoning that support their attainment. Second, the requirement to 'demonstrate' success to stakeholders of various kinds including regulators, purchasers, etc., serves to limit the scope for contested or ambivalent appraisals as far as the official face or self-consciousness of institutions is concerned. Put simply, institutions often concentrate on what they have to count (even though it is well known that 'what counts' and what can be counted are not always the same thing)[3], and in so doing they have a need to make themselves look good. These two factors come together in the value-washed language of 'performance', 'standards', 'effectiveness', or 'quality', etc. There is a whole lexicon of managerialist language which conveys the sense that what is being sought or achieved is 'a good thing' but which does so partly by ironing out complexities and contests about what patterns of health-related goods ought to be sought or achieved.

To the extent that these managerialist elements are influential within a health system there is a systemic tendency for the system and its institutions to make fundamentally important value judgements blindly or at least in obscured or disguised ways. Dominant assumptions about, or models of, healthcare can simply be structured into, and reinforced by, the managerialist preoccupation with effectiveness. In the next section I will use the example of evidence-based healthcare to illustrate this claim, and hence some of the potential value effects of managerialism, in more detail. But before doing so I think it is worth raising some very general concerns about the ethical implications of managerialism.

---

[3] An expression of this sort is sometimes attributed to Albert Einstein.

As I have characterized it here managerialism represents something of a threat to healthcare ethics and, by the same token, a possible constraint upon aspects of democratic accountability in health policy. That is to say if healthcare ethics entails an open, deliberative, and broadly based discussion about healthcare goods, then the tendencies summarized above work against such a discussion. They do so both by institutionally privileging comparatively narrow consequence-based forms of reasoning, and by doing so under a blanket of unproblematized quality speak.[4] These two tendencies have to some extent become part of the internal and external 'public relations' of institutions and are underpinned by a more or less vigorous 'hard sell'. This climate literally dampens down the agendas of healthcare ethics.

Discourses around 'value for money' or 'standards', etc. have a strong purchase on healthcare thinking and practices. They have a bewitching quality, standing as they do, for what 'commonsense' tells us can only be good. What is needed, I would suggest, is for those working in healthcare ethics to lend their weight to currents of critical reflexivity in the struggle against narrower forms of managerial reflexivity. I would want to propose the analogous argument with regard to this theme as I did in relation to inequalities in health. Namely that the more we can build literacy, and a wider self-consciousness, about the heavily value-laden processes of managerialism, the more we spread the responsibility for whatever is done through these processes.

The rise in managerialism provides an excellent example of the need for healthcare ethics to focus on the social embodiment of healthcare agency and values, and not simply upon abstract dilemmas that might face idealized 'policy-makers' or 'professionals'. Understanding the changing role of management on the value field of healthcare helps us to appreciate (a) the importance of forms of collective and dispersed agency in shaping what gets done and what gets valued; (b) the extent to which such agency and its policy effects are constituted by structural and discursive processes rather than self-conscious choices; and (c) the potential for some of these broad policy or cultural processes to positively obscure the value judgements that they are socially embedding.

I would not want a focus on structural and discursive processes to completely displace attention from management ethics as being about the choices and dilemmas facing individual managers, i.e. the differences that individuals or small groups of individuals can make in relation not only to specific cases but also to institutional norms. However, whatever the balance in our

---

[4] It is the combination of these two factors that is most problematic, an increase in the relative influence of consequentialist reasoning within healthcare cultures may, in many respects, survive critical scrutiny, however for it to do so it first has to be subject to critical scrutiny.

analysis between process and agency, management must not be understood merely as a factor that influences healthcare ethics through its impact upon health professionals' clinical roles and priorities. Management itself also represents a legitimate, and fundamentally important, locus for practical and analytical ethics. The goals, obligations, and 'comportment' of health-care institutions (for which managers are in large measure responsible) are certainly as important, and as worthy of study, as other aspects of health-professional activity. What is more, as I am seeking to illustrate, to under-stand or appraise the latter we need to understand the potential tensions between aspects of institutional ethics on the one hand and professional ethics on the other.

Managing Evidence-Based Healthcare

I will use the example of evidence-based healthcare to illustrate some of the interactions between management and healthcare ethics. Evidence-based healthcare (EBH) (or evidence-based medicine (EBM)) is a good example of the many reforming discourses which are helping to reconfigure healthcare policies and practices and which, thereby, reshape or constrain institutional and professional norms. It also shares in common with all of these 'influen-tial notions' a measure of ambiguity or, more precisely, a certain degree of interpretive elasticity, noticeable, for instance, in the gaps between what these ideas can represent 'in principle' and their embodiment 'in practice'. It is a common feature of health-policy debate to see some influential notion defended along the following lines. 'But this is only how it's been interpreted here and it doesn't need to be interpreted like that.' One of the things I want to argue in this section is that, whilst accepting that this can be a legitimate way of defending ideas, we should be somewhat suspicious of this sort of argumentative manoeuvre. EBH, if it is to be something more than a set of ideas, has to be enacted, and in the process of enactment it will be interpreted and realized in specific ways. In broad terms the nature of EBH will depend upon how it is 'managed'. To understand or evaluate EBH (including its relevance to healthcare ethics) we need to address the ways in which it is (or might be) socially realized and not just what it stands for in the abstract.

Dickenson and Vineis (2002) make a helpful distinction between what they call 'bedside EBM' and 'regulatory EBM', a distinction which illuminates the principle–practice tension that I have just introduced. Bedside EBM reflects Sackett's definition of EBM as 'the conscientious, explicit and judicious use of current best evidence in making decisions about the care of individual pa-tients', which 'integrates the best evidence with individual clinical expertise and patients' choice' (Sackett *et al.*, 1996). Dickenson and Vineis describe regulatory EBM, by contrast, as about 'the production of clinical guidelines that are meant to rationalize clinical practice but also to control medical expenditure' (2002, p. 243). This distinction can be read in a number of ways. We can see it as distinguishing between unconstrained individual professional–client relationships on the one hand and the institutional and policy constraints that inhibit professional and patient autonomy on the other. We can see it as distinguishing between a 'pure' concern with deploying evidence on the one hand and the 'smuggling in' of a very different concern with cost control. Finally, I suggest, we can see it as representing the distinction between what EBM might represent in principle and what, in many cases, it has become in practice. However, I would also want to suggest that all of these distinctions break down on closer inspection and that any attempt to locate 'the good' in bedside EBM and 'the bad' in regulatory EBM will not work (a point that Dickenson and Veneis are themselves anxious to drive home).

The limitation of a definition such as Sackett's is that it is so clearly a rationalization, indeed an idealization. It is not just that it stipulates that 'best evidence' will be used 'conscientiously' and 'judiciously' but also that this use will incorporate and be compatible with the individual expertise of doctors and the choices of individual patients. All kinds of potential problems of interpretation or conflicts of perspective are smoothed over by definitional fiat. This is acceptable, indeed may be desirable, in an idealization but it does not get us very far in practice. In practice we need to have some notion of how EBH judgements will be made and what they will look like. And, when we move to the world of practice, one thing is clear—these judgements will inevitably be open to a degree of social appraisal and social coordination. We cannot say that EBH is whatever individual health professionals say it is. For that reason EBH will necessarily manifest itself in relation to some degree of regulatory thinking, although this may be more or less weak or circumscribed. At minimum 'best evidence' is something which, given the nature of scientific evidence, has to be negotiated and (to some degree) settled socially; and once ideas about best evidence are in place professional colleagues and healthcare institutions cannot be indifferent about individual practices that appear to ignore evidence, otherwise they will share in any resulting culpability.

Hence, to restate what I said above, if we want to evaluate EBH we must ask about the ways in which it can be enacted. How do, or might, 'managers' (whether or not they are themselves also health professionals) make use of, or implement, EBH? How does management help to bring about the various 'good things' and 'bad things' that are associated with bedside or regulatory EBM?

Part of the answer to these questions was provided in the previous section. Namely the systems of target-setting, quality control, surveillance, or performance management which make up the core of managerialism are very closely allied to the regulatory role of EBH. The discourses of performance management and of EBH are certainly different but (a) there are striking affinities between their underlying rationalities and purposes and (b) they can be, and often are, intertwined in practice. The 'lenses' of surveillance and the tools of what has come to be called 'clinical governance' are to a large extent informed by, and of course legitimated by 1 reference to EBH.

I say 'legitimated' because the language of 'best evidence' promises to add a good measure of rigour and robustness to what might otherwise seem like the vagaries of managerial decision-making. The functions of clinical governance include weeding out practices that do patients more harm than good, limiting practices that have no demonstrable benefit, and guiding practitioners in the direction of practices which stand the most chance of benefiting their patients. Expressed in these broad terms these are clearly valuable functions and functions that illustrate the major potential benefits of EBH. They also, incidentally, show the inextricable link, in practice, between a concern with effectiveness and a concern with cost-effectiveness. The only reason to limit well-meaning, apparently harmless, but also benefit-less practices is that they depend upon finite human and other resources which might be directed at some good. Indeed, a focus on costs is not something alien smuggled into EBH. Evidence-based methods work at least as well in relation to questions of costs as they do in relation to questions of effectiveness. (This is not to deny that there are sensible worries about the way cost-effectiveness judgements can work in EBH, as I will indicate below.)

Managers can, therefore, deploy the lessons of EBH through methods of clinical governance in order to promote and underpin effective (and cost-effective) working within their institutions. They may do this more or less self-consciously and independently. But in large measure the form and content of clinical-governance methods will be shaped outside of particular institutions and will be disseminated by powerful agencies who, to some degree, 'manage' the managers.

It is the combination of factors that I have rehearsed so far that gives rise to what I would argue are the key issues of management ethics with regard to EBH. That is, given that EBH: (i) can be directed at very worthwhile ends, (ii) plays a legitimating function because of its claims to rigour and robustness, and (iii) through the way it is embedded in systems and methods of clinical governance, is routinely transmitted through the cultures and practices of healthcare institutions, how can managers maintain some degree of scepticism about its possible uses and effects? What, in fact, can managers do to ensure that the effects of EBH on clinical practice are ethically defensible? I cannot pretend to answer these questions here but there is certainly a need for managers to take these questions, and the issues they represent, seriously. It is very important to build a shared understanding within the community of healthcare managers and practitioners and not just amongst commentators that in practice EBH is not always and everywhere or necessarily 'a good thing'. This understanding depends upon the recognition that EBH is not a value-neutral activity but rather is an activity that carries specific value-sets, and shapes healthcare according to these value-sets; and, depending upon contexts and cases, that these value-sets need to be interrogated (e.g. see Frith, 2002).[5]

Dickenson and Vineis (2002) pull together the major potential value-effects of EBH, and the ways in which these can be a source of concern with regard to both the quality and ethics of healthcare. Here I will summarize these effects before reflecting on the scope for managers to take them into account. In brief their argument is that models of research and evidence necessarily have certain values built into them (a phenomenon which others have labelled 'implicit normativity' (Molewijk *et al.*, 2003)). This is so both because of the kinds of measures used (for example, how far do measures focus on the 'relative benefit' or on the 'population-attributable benefit' of treatments?) and because the needed measurements require us to abstract out, and focus upon, only specific kinds of 'inputs' and 'outputs' from the whole healthcare process. As a result these approaches inevitably favour certain kinds of services and treatments over others (those most suited to these models of research). Thus, generally speaking, drug trials are likely to lend themselves to the models of EBH more easily than small-scale experiments in surgery, and both of these things will have some advantages over innovations in specialist psychosocial nursing interventions, where positivistic methods of measurement and research may seem out of place.

An important product of this implicit normativity is that EBH measures can systematically disadvantage certain groups, such as particular groups of elderly people or people with chronic illnesses, for example, in those cases where there is some, but only comparatively limited, evidence of suitably demonstrable *effectiveness* of the treatments in questions. Also, and at the same time, EBH-related policies can and do support rationing systems with similar effects, and take these rationing choices out of the hands of professionals, because of their potential to compare, and produce 'authoritative' judgements about the general *cost-effectiveness* of treatments. The combined side effects of these policies, therefore, can be not only to constrain profes-

---

[5] It is important to stress that acknowledging the value-laden nature of EBH is no reason to abandon it as a project and does not negate the important contribution that it can make to planning and delivering healthcare. It is merely to acknowledge that EBH, in being value-laden, is no different from any other social phenomenon: in the case of some social phenomena this characteristic is obvious, whereas with others, such as EBH, it is positively disguised. Managers are, therefore, not in a position to 'safeguard' EBH from being value-laden, but they are in a position not only to be reflexive about the way EBH shapes healthcare values but also, in many instances, to affect those shaping processes.

sional and therapeutic autonomy but, by so doing, undermine the flexibility of health professionals to be responsive to individuals in the way person-centred care philosophies demand. In other words EBH-related policies can contribute significantly to the two trends I introduced in Chapter 7: the shift from substantive to technical rationalities, and the shift towards institutional agency at the expense of more independent individual agency.

Although, as I have said, many of these value-effects will be produced and transmitted from outside particular institutions there is, even within institutions, some scope for both (a) how the governance measures that are informed by EBH are interpreted and enacted in particular sites, i.e. how flexibly imaginatively and judiciously forms of regulation or control are applied and (b) greater transparency and critical self-consciousness about the decision-making and the particular judgements which make up the local regime of governance. These forms of appraisal can and should take place at every level, from the system level, through to particular cases in particular contexts. Critical appraisal cannot eliminate ethically contentious judgements nor reconcile ethical balancing acts. These are inevitable. But what it can do is to minimize the chance of such judgements or balancing acts being 'decided' blindly, hidden behind the plausible reassurance offered by the discourses of EBH.

Management, the Patient, and Society

In the remainder of the chapter I will attempt to summarize and review the effects of the rise of health-service management on the value field of health-care and healthcare ethics. To do so I will necessarily be dealing with broad trends and making some (to some degree unwarranted) generalizations, but I hope, nonetheless, that this is a worthwhile task. As the example of EBH illustrates, one way in which the management role has been represented in recent healthcare-ethics literature is as 'coming between' the health profes-sional and the patient (see discussions in Khushf, 2000 and Wong, 2000). Managerial mechanisms-such as the ones discussed above, including tightly defined budgets, formularies, guidelines and protocols, published perform-ance indicators, financial incentive systems-structure and 'interfere with' what would otherwise be a comparatively 'pure' professional–patient en-counter. To put it in these terms is to exaggerate but it makes the point. Of course in reality there have never been purely idealistic and altruistic profes-sional–patient relationships. All such relationships exist in a world of mixed motives and practical compromise. (I explore this in more depth in the next chapter.) But traditional models of healthcare professionalism stress the intrinsic and vocational properties of the relationship in which the professional acts in the best interests of the patient and the patient trusts the professional to do so. This traditional stress on the beneficent and fiduciary elements of the professional–patient relationship is independent of whether professional or patient autonomy is foregrounded in the model of professionalism. It arises because healthcare relationships are often unequal in relation to knowledge and personal vulnerability, and, however economically independent and powerful patients are, they need to be able to trust that the professional will act in their best interests. Managerial mechanisms seen in this light undermine the autonomy of the professional to decide, unhindered, on what is best for the patient, and undermine the confidence of the patient that this is what is being done.

However, as I have tried to show, this largely negative reading of the influence of health-service management is insufficient. As the pharmacy example in the last chapter indicated, when we focus in on a specific mechanism our appraisals of its effects becomes more balanced, and depend a great deal on whose interests we focus upon. From the point of view of an individual patient a particular mechanism may be unfortunate but it may, in other respects, benefit a group of patients as a whole. Similarly restricting the exercise of professional autonomy in some respects may enhance the scope for autonomous choice amongst a wider group of professionals within an institution. In fact, the strong emphasis on individual professional autonomy and discretion in traditional models of health professionalism only ever applied to certain occupational roles, particularly doctors, in the first place. Other occupational roles, particularly nurses, have always been better viewed as part of a managed service (Norman and Cowley, 1998), collectively organized to fulfil tasks defined in large part by others.

In order to assess the ethical implications of new patterns of health-service management we need to adopt the multilevel analysis I have discussed elsewhere. In relation both to specific managerial mechanisms and to the ways in which these mechanisms work in clusters (their compound structural and discursive effects) we need to examine the ethical defensibility of the policy-making that creates them, their overall effects on the experience and distribution of health-related goods, and as only one part of this process their specific effects on models of professionalism and responsiveness to patients. I should underline that I would not expect to come to one singular conclusion about the ethical effects of health-service management. Indeed, I am assuming that the management of health professionals is a necessity in some shape or form. Of course certain management mechanisms, in certain contexts, will withstand much closer ethical scrutiny than others. For example, it is difficult to see how a healthcare institution could justify paying doctors personal rewards in direct compensation for them avoiding the prescription of very expensive drugs, although this could be, in some respects, a 'cost-effective' strategy. On the other hand, pharmaceutical-surveillance systems which monitor the 'over prescription' of certain drugs, e.g. antibiotics, and provide some institutional rewards for low levels of over-prescription may well be perfectly defensible.

I am suggesting that behind all of the complexity and diversity of the mechanisms it deploys health-service management serves, amongst other things, to balance individual interests and population interests. It is for this reason that health-service management is of central relevance to a book about the social context of healthcare ethics and the tension between population-oriented and patient-oriented perspectives. Certainly the exact function of management systems, and the conception of the relevant population to serve, depends upon the nature of the health polity and the organizing principles of the healthcare system. In a market model the population may, in the first instance, only be fellow contributors to the same scheme. In a welfare-state model the population may represent all citizens (or anyone who falls within the defined welfare net). Nevertheless there are some strong commonalities here even between these two ideal type positions, and these commonalities are greater still once we acknowledge the much more 'mixed' health polities that exist in practice.

Of course doctors and other health professionals have always had to find ways of balancing the interests of specific patients and wider populations. This is what is at stake in ethical dilemmas about confidentiality in cases of potentially dangerous or highly infectious individuals. Everyone has some obligation to consider the effects of their actions on the public good and health professionals also have specific roles and responsibilities in relation to public health (which I will consider in the next chapter). Similarly it has often been pointed out that doctors, for example, need to make decisions about how best to divide their time between patients in a queue, or how to divide their time between patient care, teaching, and research, and in so doing are de facto weighing specific patient claims against more general claims. Keown's (1994) account of the grounds of professional ethics, for instance, takes as one of its themes this tension between the duties of the professional to their client and their broader duties to serve the 'good' (justice, health, etc.) they profess to serve. But it is also striking that Keown, in company with many other theorists of professionalism, stresses first and foremost the special nature of the individual doctor–patient relationship, and the conditions of mutual trust which it is meant to reflect and support. The background assumption behind this kind of account, sometimes stated explicitly, is that within certain side constraints, the doctor's role is to serve the immediate patient's best interests. There may be specific circumstances in which this creates a dilemma for the doctor, but normally it will not do so.

This assumption of strong patient-centredness has, as discussed in Chapter 3, been elevated into an ideal or ideology in various ways. It is, if you like, a 'useful myth'[6] for both patients and doctors to embrace. In its boldest form, the notion that the professional will do whatever is best for the patient (somehow determined), it obviously collides with some immediate real-world complications. It assumes that the professional team are in a position to make available whatever time and resources the patient may benefit from (or need, depending on the conception of 'best'). Most models of healthcare funding mean that this ideal-type assumption has to be qualified considerably. And even a fee-for-service model, which only the few could afford on a regular basis, entails that the patient can only get what is best so far as their purse allows. Hence a focus on health-service management highlights tensions which otherwise are seen to lie in the background of healthcare ethics, and which the myth of strong patient-centredness constructs as marginal ones but which are perhaps better seen as pervasive ones. Having said that, however, there are real risks that certain approaches to health-service management may exacerbate the tensions in, and undermine some of the assumptions of, healthcare professionalism, in precisely the ways critics of 'managed care' fear. Making this judgement requires a closer examination of the impact of management mechanisms on the value field of healthcare.

The question that needs closest attention here is the extent to which, and the manner in which, some forms of managerialism colonize and reconstruct healthcare-professional subjectivities and practices. I am thinking here of the kinds of mechanisms mentioned above, guidelines, performance indicators, formularies, etc., which have grown in the wake of a broader societal interest in both resource stewardship and professional accountability. These mechanisms are built into more or less strict and tangible institutional norms either directly or indirectly. That is, on the one hand an institution might establish an explicit norm, and monitor or regulate adherence to it to varying degrees, or on the other hand personal and institutional incentive structures may construct more or less unspoken norms of behaviour and practice evaluation. In the first case, for example, the relevant institution's indications for the availability of treatment types may be defined. In the second case, for example, the factors which appear in published league tables may become central to the micro-allocation of effort whereas other, arguably equally important factors, may be relatively neglected. But in both cases norms are established which structure professional work and enter into professional subjectivity to some degree. These mechanisms, in many instances, serve to increase the influence of more generic and impersonal norms in healthcare, not only at the institutional level where impersonal standards, measures, and priorities have a natural place but also at the level of the individual professional–patient encounter where their place is more contestable.

---

[6] I do not wish to assert that what I am calling 'myths' are falsehoods. I am simply leaving aside questions about the extent to which elements of them can be said to be true.

Institutional norms of this kind always pose a potential threat to the scope of professional autonomy, flexibility, and responsiveness. Of course in some cases they may simply safeguard a patient's best interests. (Where, for example, x intervention has been shown to be simply not suitable for condition y, and doctors are denied the clinical freedom to do x for y.) But, very often, these norms create a conflict between a person-centred perspective and institutional goals, and between vocational and institutional identities. The professional is faced with a generic, impersonal framework on the one hand and the specificity of the case in front of them on the other, the unique combination of clinical, personal, and social conditions of the patient plus the patient's specific wishes and values. Their professional identity has to accommodate both their loyalty to the specific patient whose interest they are there to protect and promote and their loyalty to the institution that provides the possibility of their work. This way of putting things brings home the point that this is not merely an interpersonal problem, a tension between professionals and managers, but an intrapersonal one, a tension between aspects of the traditional professional–client relationship and accepted managerial norms. (We are, as it is sometimes put, all managers now.)

Before trying to draw together the threads of this chapter I want to stress again that I think there is no unequivocal way of judging the ethical defensibility of, and effects of, health-service management. No doubt some management practices could be judged to be simply unacceptable because they produce clearly bad outcomes or embody a profound lack of respect for professionals or patients, but more typically the kinds of mechanisms being discussed here have both things to recommend them *and* things to make us sceptical about them. And where we place the emphasis is dependent upon whose perspective we adopt and on our underlying models of the health system and health professionalism. To summarize, and somewhat simplify, these mechanisms often have the effect of shifting the orientation of health services from individual agendas towards social agendas. The extent to which we think this is a good thing depends upon how far we think this is desirable and possible (and of course how well the mechanisms work), and all of this in turn partly depends upon what we think healthcare systems are for. I will try to specify the core issues more carefully in the final section of this chapter, and then explore them further in Chapter 9.

The Ethics of Managed Health Professionalism

In saying that management mechanisms tend to represent a shift from an individual towards a social orientation I am pulling together three distinct, although overlapping, shifts in emphasis. Namely: the shift from individual towards social goals; the shift from person-specific towards generic evaluative frameworks; and the shift from 'professional partiality' towards greater impartiality. Particular mechanisms will combine these features to varying degrees. The first is the most general in nature, and simply represents the fact that institutions and systems meet collective ends as well as individual ends, and there will be times when these things do not completely coincide. A collective end may be to reduce the incidence of an infectious disease, and this may require a greater level of compliance with treatment than an individual would choose. It may be gathering epidemiological data in ways that entail a lower threshold of consent to testing than some individuals are happy with. It might, of course, include more abstract collective ends related to efficiency, equity, or solidarity, etc. The second shift relates, for example, to the use of less fine-grained decision frameworks. A formulary embodies this shift when it rules out certain treatments which may be ideal for particular individuals in favour of others which are perhaps adequate but allow less person-specific prescription. Enforced protocols and guidelines produce the same effect and the coarser frameworks they employ entail a reductionism in practice. Healthcare becomes less tailored to unique patients who have to accept more 'off the peg' responses. (It is the combination of these two shifts in emphasis which I am suggesting is particularly important and which provides the rationale for this book.) To the extent that various conceptions of 'social goods' are built into the explicit or implicit evaluative frameworks of healthcare decision-making then the value field of healthcare professional ethics evolves in what I am calling a 'population-oriented' direction. The third shift is the most difficult to state or evaluate. I will discuss it more fully.

Health professionals have always placed an emphasis upon impartiality in their dealings with others. This is a central feature of the ideology of professionalism. A professional, or at least a professional with a concern for ethical integrity, would not want to treat someone differently because of irrelevant characteristics—race, class, or gender for example. Nor would they want to divide their time and attention between people in ways that reflect these kinds of characteristics. Similarly, faced with a dispute between two or more of their patients they would no doubt endeavour to be fair to all parties. However, the tradition of patient-centredness, as well as representing the importance of patient-specificity, also represents an element of patient advocacy. Health professionals work, in certain respects, on behalf of their patients, and have specific obligations to their patients that they do not have to other people. Although the impartiality of health professionals between patients ought not to be in doubt, it becomes more complicated if we ask about whether health professionals ought to be impartial between patients and non-patients. Within the health system (and sometimes within the wider society) the doctor or nurse is sometimes the representative of their patient and their patient's interests.

This point can be expressed in different ways. We could say that impartial systems require that patients have representatives who to some extent 'take their side', for example in tussles about resource allocation. This does not mean that the professional is being 'partial', rather they are acting as a representative for the sake of global impartiality. (This is the model of legal advocacy of course.) But we might just as well say that global impartiality requires some circumscribed forms of partiality at the level of the individual professional. And, although professional partiality has a different affective character than that amongst family and friends there are many cases in which it is quite strongly analogous, for example, where a doctor or nurse has worked closely with a family through the long course of a chronic illness. What is more, if we believe, as seems plausible, that these kinds of personal closeness, 'moderated love' (Campbell, 1984), or affective engagement, are sometimes intrinsic to good healthcare, then we might prefer to talk openly about partiality so as to acknowledge this analogy with other special relationships. It is in this sense that management mechanisms which play up collective ends and impersonal norms can be seen also as a shift in emphasis away from what I have called professional partiality.

These three shifts, albeit only in emphasis, between patient orientations and social orientations, brought about by increasing health-service managerialism, constitute one of the major recent movements in the social construction of healthcare-professional roles. Within the health systems and institutions affected they amount to a significant change in the definition of and division of health work, from person-centredness towards greater population-centredness, with the latter orientation being more fully embodied in many more roles. To the extent that these changes bite into reality, doctor–patient relationships, in particular, are reconstructed. Those doctors who complain about managed-care approaches are right to question their impact on traditional definitions of professionalism, although perhaps sometimes too quick to condemn changes which are multifaceted and ethically ambiguous. A proper assessment requires an integrated evaluation of system-level goals, the styles of responsibilization embedded in specific managerial regimes, and their effects on professional–patient relationships. At each of these levels there are a range of philosophical challenges. We need, most generally speaking, to be able to understand both (a) the proper balance between the public good and person-centredness, including professional partiality, in the construction of healthcare, and (b) the policy, institutional and practical mechanisms which might best achieve this balance within specific health systems.

9

The Boundaries of Professional Legitimacy

Encounters between professionals and clients change as healthcare and health systems evolve. The various impacts of managerialism, discussed in the last chapter, are one way in which the 'rules of the game' change, but these impacts overlap with, and are sometimes a product of, the broader set of changes that I have called the diffusion of the health agenda. In this chapter I want to consider the effects of some of these broader changes, especially the greater involvement of health professionals in health promotion, for the 'rules of the game' in professional–patient encounters. In summary my argument is that these changes are broadly analogous to those associated with managerialism, and that they have important implications for healthcare-professional ethics as well as for health education and health policy more broadly, implications which will be discussed in the final part of the book.

As I mentioned in the Preface one way of summarizing the nature of the issues I am reviewing here is to see them as representing the convergence of currents in the sociology of the health professions with currents in healthcare ethics. Sociology, by its very nature, is concerned to 'see beyond' the self-understandings of health professionals, about their purposes and rationales, to the wider social processes which are embodied and reproduced in health work. A sociological understanding has to be able to encompass both first-person accounts of what actions are meant to achieve and wider readings of what is actually accomplished by the social practices of which the actions are a part. Those healthcare ethicists who have been exercised about the reconfiguration of professional ethics by changes such as managed care are wrestling with a very similar problem. They are interested in the internal evaluation of healthcare practices and they are also interested in the ways in which these practices, seen more broadly, are accomplishing social agendas such as cost containment or professional regulation.

Explanations of the rise in prominence of healthcare ethics or new ethical agendas often point to key material factors such as new technological possibilities, or resource pressures. These kinds of explanations have a role to play but, as I noted in Part I, it is also necessary to consider broader and more diffuse social changes including changes in the importance, bases, and forms of professional power and changes in conceptions of healthcare goods. In what follows I am taking the increasing influence of the language of health promotion as representative of some of these changes. When a doctor and patient meet in an era of health promotion the nature of the encounter has changed, and their individual and shared expectations about the purposes and the mode of the encounter have 'moved on' correspondingly, although not always of course in exactly the same way. In this chapter I will reflect on the ways in which a number of elements of health promotion, namely its prevention orientation, its population orientation, and its well-being orientation, shape professional–patient relationships and also consider their compound effects.

An Imperative to Screen?

One element of health promotion is the shift in emphasis it entails from treatment towards prevention. This carries with it a new kind of future orientation, and the associated readiness of health professionals to construct their client's 'health needs' against a longer time-frame. The 'health promotion mind-set' places the patient's immediate concerns and demands against the background of the possibility of them living as long and healthy a life as possible. This can lead to an increase in the gap between professional and patient perspectives. Here is just one example, again, drawn from routine practice.

Debbie, a woman general practitioner (GP), has spent most of the 15 minutes she gave over to a consultation with a young female patient, Bridget, to discussing Bridget's failure to turn up for cervical screening pap smear tests. Debbie is a little concerned about the disruption to the appointments system but is mainly worried about Bridget's future health and her reluctance to comply with the screening programme. Debbie is a strong believer in the value of the cervical screening programme and the importance of her patient's participation in it, and she believes also, with sincerely beneficient intent, that time talking with Bridget may help to 'uncover' Bridget's perceptions and motivations, and ultimately help to change them. At the back of Debbie's mind are some niggles about whether she has made the best use of the consultation time but generally she believes that she has done the best she can.

In this case it is clear that there is a significant gap between Debbie and Bridget. It is quite possible, for example, that from Bridget's perspective the doctor's interest seems unwelcome and intrusive. It is equally possible that Bridget feels that the factors and reasons which took her into the consultation in the first place have been largely ignored or dismissed. The doctor's genuine orientation towards the prevention of future possible harms may not be shared by the patient, and may add to already existing conflicts of perspective. This example thereby also serves to illustrate the ever-increasing 'strain' on the consultation which, amongst many other things, has to incorporate multiple elements of the future as well as the present and the past. One of the things at stake in this encounter is the doctor trying to draw the patient into the arena of health promotion, trying to 'spread' the health promotion mind-set to the patient. (Of course patients may equally well be trying to draw the doctor into their agendas but are often less well placed to do so, depending upon the settings, conventions, and power relationships inherent in the meeting.)

In this sort of case Bridget may well feel that the 'rules of the game' are other than those she was expecting. She visited the doctor, let us suppose, for advice about a swollen ankle, caused by a domestic accident, which has affected her mobility. But this is dealt with very quickly by some 'reassurance' that it looks OK, by the advice to 'wait and see' for a few days, and by the promise of treatment if and when it is needed. Bridget arrives at the clinic ready to talk about all of these things, and also anxious about how she is going to manage her job under the circumstances and vaguely wondering if she should ask for a 'sick note' to authorize her entitlement to paid sick leave. She arrives preoccupied with one set of issues relating to her immediate needs but she finds herself being pressed to talk about other things, things that she does not really want to talk about, and which do not meet her felt needs.

This case also has to be considered alongside those of Debbie's other patients for whom the need for this conversation does not arise because they cooperate with the demands of the screening programme. Bridget's non-compliance makes her relationship to the screening programme highly visible, but of course all the other women who fall within the remit of the programme have also been subject to processes of programme inclusion of one sort or another. The fact that these other women have gone along with the programme more or less willingly and may be happy to see it as a good thing, does not mean that Debbie is not implicated in processes of social regulation which bring about the 'success' of the programme. In the case of Bridget the intervention and the change in the nature of the professional–patient encounter is conspicuous, in the case of the other women much less so, but in all cases they are equally real. For Bridget, and for the other women in different ways, it is reasonable to ask whether the doctor's involvement with this screening programme changes the basis of the professional–patient relationship enough to cast doubt on it. The changes here seem broadly equivalent to those considered in relation to managed care which are said to potentially undermine the fiduciary model of the relationship. The doctor, it could be said, is not simply responding to the interests of the individual patient but is importing other, possibly incompatible, values and imperatives into the relationship. In this situation why should the patient trust the professional, indeed is there not reason to worry that the trust which has been earned on one set of assumptions is being misused because those assumptions no longer apply?

To begin to explore these questions I want to first consider some of the possible (conscious or unconscious) motivations behind Debbie's encounter with Bridget. For the sake of argument I will separate out three kinds of motivation. (1) Debbie is concerned with her patient's well-being and believes that screening can contribute to it; she also has a strong sense of fairness and knows that it is often those who most need interventions who do not receive them, this has built up in her a disposition to invest effort in 'hard-to-get' patients and this is the habit which is enacted with Bridget. (2) Debbie understands that the success of the screening programme, considered as a whole, depends upon a high uptake of screening. Below a certain level of uptake the population benefits are quite small for the large cost of the screening-service provision. Although she knows that the chance of the service being of benefit to any single individual is quite small, she aims to get more than 90 per cent uptake and this means from time to time investing time in 'selling' the screening to certain individuals. (3) Debbie's practice has a target of 90 per cent uptake, set because this protects the cost effectiveness of the service. If this target is met then significant financial bonuses are paid to the practice.

The first motivation relates to the perceived best interests of the patient, the second to the needs of the service and the population it serves, and the third adds to this the interests of the doctors concerned (this might be their own personal financial interests or the interests of the institution they work for and all those, including patients, who are affected by it). In reality it is quite possible that all of these factors are relevant. The first kind of motivation stays close to the basis of the ideal type fiduciary model. It is always possible that doctors' and patients' conceptions of best interests can vary, the different emphasis placed upon the salience of screening can be seen simply as one instance of this. The third kind of motivation is that provided by the kind of managerial mechanisms discussed in the last chapter. But it can be seen that the second kind of motivation might produce very similar effects to this without the support of overt incentives. The population orientation of health-promotion work can insert itself into the individual professional–patient relationship independently of specific management pressures or incentive systems.

The above example serves to introduce some of the interests and influences which shape professional–patient encounters. As well as the interests of the doctors and patients involved there are also, in this case, the interests of all those with a stake in population-orientated services. It also serves as a reminder of some of the more subtle forms of influence in play in healthcare relationships. Some of the forms of social regulation represented by the cervical-screening case are almost invisible and can perhaps best be seen through the Foucauldian notion of 'disciplinary power' introduced in Chapter 2 which is often used by sociologists to criticize health promotion. Systems of health screening, endorsed and delivered by health professionals, play their part in the construction of normative systems. These normative systems around health promotion produce types of health-related self-consciousness and self-surveillance, and thereby new forms of subjectivity and identity that have been labelled 'health-promoting subjects' (Bunton *et al.*, 1995). Individuals, that is, who take it for granted that they should be looking after their health and that this requires participation in health-promoting practices such as these programmes. From this perspective doctors are only one node in, and medium for, the spread of the health-promotion mind-set. They are themselves as much a product of the health-promotion discourses that they reproduce as their patients.

However, cervical screening, although future-oriented and population-oriented, still represents a fairly tightly framed and recognizable healthcare intervention. In the next section I will briefly consider other actual or potential shifts in the rules of the game which derive from concerns with 'positive health'.

Reforming Lives

Here is another quick example just to open up the issues further. Suppose our doctor, Debbie, is looking after John. John has had 'lifestyle' screening for heart-disease risk factors. Debbie is considering prescribing a statin for their cholesterol-lowering effects but she is wary of simply looking for a medical solution. She believes John's entire lifestyle also needs a rethink. He should be aiming for a better 'work/life balance', living a less sedentary lifestyle, eating a more balanced diet including less fat, giving up smoking, learning to relax more, and finding leisure-time projects and interests to give him some sense of fulfilment outside of his job. Debbie and her team have many patients who fall into a category such as this. People whose health and lives are being impaired by their lifestyle and for whom what they really want to prescribe is lifestyle reform. Now it is important that I do not suggest that this is a new thing; doctors and other healers have always had this involvement with lifestyles as well as specific illness. It is merely that the growth in health promotion as a self-conscious movement draws attention to tensions between this lifestyle-reform role and the relatively narrow forms of clinical knowledge which are the main foundation of health-professional authority in the modern world. In a climate where there is already widespread scepticism about potential abuses of professional authority there is a sharper awareness of the proper scope and limits of that authority. Let us imagine that Debbie herself is self-conscious about these matters. She wants to explore ways of confronting John about his lifestyle but she is unsure what exactly it is legitimate for her to do. Prescribing the statins, with his informed consent, is relatively straightforward. Although having to take tablets has the effect of making him see himself as 'sick' in some respects, he is happy to accept the authority of the doctor that he is 'at risk' and that this is an appropriate response to the risk. It is precisely the ability to deploy the discourses and practices of the sick role which enable this to be a smooth transaction. Talking about exercise and diet and giving advice about possible changes and perhaps referral to specialist sources of advice and support is also comparatively easy, although Debbie is conscious that this might create something of a judgemental feel to the consultation. The territory here is less medical and more a question of the way John 'chooses' to live his life. It thus becomes more difficult for both parties to 'hide behind' the sick role, and the issues become contested in a different way, i.e. they are much more about conflicts in personal values and beliefs than uncertain clinical science.

This is more evident still in connection with questions like work/life balance, leisure-time projects, and relaxation. Should Debbie, or one of her colleagues, encourage John to get back to reading novels, which he has got out of the habit of doing? Perhaps they could or should recommend certain novels to him or even make them available to him, or refer him to a local book group? It is obvious where this is going. There are countless ways in which the healthcare team might like to gently intervene in John's life. Thus far they are all predicated on preventive healthcare but they need not be. Debbie may be of the opinion that the statins are the most evidence-based method of reducing risks for John but also concerned about what she feels is, based on his accounts, his poor quality of life. Her job, as she sees it, is to look after John holistically and to help him live a life that he feels, or could come to feel, is fuller, more worthwhile, and more contented. She is interested in his 'positive health'. But, as these examples suggest and as I discussed in Chapter 2, there is no clear way of drawing lines between 'positive health' and other aspects of well-being. Hence there is no decisive way of drawing boundaries around a health professional's legitimate scope of intervention on the one hand and unwarranted intrusion on the other. If John turned up at the surgery to be regaled with advice or encouragement about his investment portfolio, his taste in girlfriends, or his rather selfish attitude to the family car he would no doubt be appalled; but why should he feel differently on hearing advice on other aspects of his lifestyle designed to improve his quality of life? He may well feel, like Bridget in the previous case, that his consultation has been hijacked by other agendas, agendas which stem from other people's interests and influences and which are, to him, unhelpful and unwelcome. He might feel this even more strongly if he knew that the practice also had screening and intervention targets for heart-disease prevention or for 'well man' counselling, and that he had been caught up by their effects.

In short all of the three major orientations of health promotion, its prevention orientation, its population orientation, and its well-being orientation, raise questions about the boundaries of professional authority and legitimacy in professional–patient encounters. They all, in different ways, also challenge widespread assumptions about the role and nature of health-related consultations.

Consultations or Interventions?

One way of approaching these assumptions is to contrast the notions of 'consultation' and 'intervention'. The former is more associated with healthcare, the latter with health promotion; the former emphasizes the agency of the patient, the latter the agency of the professional. As ever it is essential to avoid over generalizing but these associations are significant. The language of consultation suggests a person-centred responsiveness, the language of intervention suggests outcome-oriented action. I want to briefly review two kinds of background assumptions about health encounters which are put in question by the rise of the health-promotion mind-set. These assumptions both relate to the centrality of the felt needs of the patient. They relate to patient expectations of health professionals as a source of support, and patient expectations about the locus of professional ends.

Patients go to health professionals looking for certain kinds of support. Thus even if clinical knowledge is the most visible underpinning for health-professional authority, the function of health-professional roles may relate more to personal support than to clinical expertise. The support which is sought is not only practical but also emotional and moral. Even in cases which are clearly disease-centred, e.g. where a patient is looking for support in managing an episode of illness or a chronic condition, the role of the consultation obviously transcends clinical-disease management. Amongst other things the patient's anxieties may need to be heard, acknowledged and thereby, to some extent, 'contained' by the professional. This is one of the things that is invoked by the idea of person-centred healthcare. As I have noted before healthcare has to incorporate care and not just health. Within nursing many theorists have argued that these kinds of caring relationships are definitive of the nursing role (see Benner and Wrubel (1989) and the discussion in Bowden (1997)). Within medicine their place is less clear-cut, but no one could deny that they have an important place. The point is that engagement with the patient as person, with the patient's subjectivity and lived experience, is an intrinsic part of healthcare. These forms of mutuality have instrumental value, they provide the professional with necessary data and provide a basis for professional influence over the patient, but they are not only instrumental, they are valuable in themselves. Indeed, these interpersonal processes are, as I have discussed earlier, part of the point of healthcare. Hence in the case described above Bridget somehow feels let down by her doctor's shift in focus; even though it is well intentioned Bridget feels as if it 'misses her out'.

The background assumption that the professional is there as a source of support is normally accompanied by the assumption, on the part of patients, that the health professionals they consult are operating within a circumscribed horizon of concerns. Partly this reflects the kinds of issues rehearsed in the cases of both Bridget and John, above, about the long-term and 'whole-life' dimensions of health promotion, where the patients are expecting shorter-term and illness-related agendas. Partly it relates to the question about the balances between patient and population orientations. As suggested above the widely shared 'traditional' background model of professional–patient encounters is that the professional is first and foremost serving the best interests (on some interpretation) of the immediate patient and not using the patient to serve some kind of other agenda or meet some broader institutional or social goal. Of course as I have also explained before this background model does not necessarily correspond to real-world health professional roles—I will say more about this in a moment—but it is certainly a model conjured up by the idea of 'consultation'.

The idea of 'intervention' has a very different feel to it. It is a more neutral and a 'blanker' notion. Above all it is an instrumental sounding idea. The health professional acts to change something about the patient or the patient's life or environment in order to bring about some end or ends. Given that the professionals are 'doing health promotion' and are acting in good faith we can take it for granted that these ends are judged, by them, to be valuable ones. But, continuing in this rather abstract and stark vein, there is nothing in the notion of a health-promotion intervention to entail that the end is seen as valuable by the patient himself or herself. Furthermore there is no reason to suppose that the valuable end even pertains to the patient. It is only fair to add at once that real-world advocates of health promotion would certainly wish to distance themselves from this picture. They would, reasonably and understandably, wish to insert values relating to consent, mutuality, and responsiveness into their models of health promotion. Nonetheless for illustrative purposes this stark picture is useful; it shows the health professional as a technologist looking for the right buttons to press to bring about the health system's desired 'health outcomes'. On this picture patients are principally objects for manipulation rather than subjects to be met with and responded to.

In reality health professionals are caught between these two ideal types of patient responsiveness and outcome-led intervention. It is unreasonable to expect the professional's concerns to be always confined by those of the patient. Not only must they be open to alternative conceptions of goods but they have other sets of obligations and relations of accountability than those arising from the immediate patient. On the other hand the patient has typically chosen to put themselves in the care of the professional and has not done so to be used as a means to an end. The tensions in play here are bound up with the fundamental ethical tensions between 'respecting values' and 'creating values' (Griffin, 1996: 61). There are obviously dangers if health professionals see themselves as something like ideal utilitarian calculators wholly focused upon 'doing as much good as possible'. But equally health professionals must have some regard for the bigger picture and not merely for their immediate patient's needs, and must take ethical responsibility for all of the implications of their choices.

What Ought Health Professionals to Do?

This ideal type contrast between consultation and intervention highlights the core concern of this chapter, what kinds of things are health professionals justified in doing? More specifically what are the proper spheres of action for health professionals, and how far ought these to be defined in relation to client expectations and the conditions for trust? I should underline the fact that in asking the question 'what ought health professionals to do?', in this context, I am not primarily asking about the self-conscious choices of health professionals. I am asking about the ways in which the roles of health professionals are constructed. My question is more about their positions in ethical space than about how they choose to operate from these positions.

The first thing to acknowledge is the wide variety of health-professional roles. This diversity was discussed in Chapter 7 as was the comparatively narrow relevance of the patient-centred consultation as a paradigm of health-care. To reiterate, health-professional roles can be population-oriented rather than individual patient-oriented; health professionals can work as part of managed teams working with groups of patients at a time e.g. many nursing roles); health professionals often have responsibilities relating primarily to systems, institutions, or procedures rather than directly to patients (e.g. management roles). In each of these cases the authorization and ethical legitimacy of these roles cannot be determined solely by reference to specific clients. In these cases the appropriate conditions for the trust of actual or potential clients may well remain a key test of legitimacy, but it is not easy to decide how to balance the importance of client trust with other possible indicators of legitimacy such as service to the public interest. The argument I am setting out in this part of the book can be summarized by saying that all health-professional roles are, in effect, like these obviously 'anomalous' cases!

To illustrate the problem of assessing the boundaries of professional legitimacy it is worth briefly considering some strongly distinctive cases where accountability conflicts are to the fore. (This is also a strategy adopted by Sorell (2001), which has influenced my thinking about this area.) For example, consider a doctor employed by the police. She might well be asked to examine and 'collect evidence' from a victim of crime. Imagine that the latter is not really keen to cooperate, but rather feels the need for more time and space. Should the doctor proceed with exactly the same mixture of support and encouragement in her police role as she might if she was simply the victim's personal doctor? Or, provided she avoids clear cut coercion would she be justified in exerting a little more persuasion and a little less responsiveness? What if the police ask her to provide them with a blood sample from an unconscious 'drink-drive' suspect? Under normal circumstances a doctor would not countenance this idea but it is put to her, as a police employee, that the blood sample must be taken soon for it to pick up the alcohol and that the driver will be allowed to give or withhold consent to the sample actually being used for a test at a later time.[1] In these instances it is clear that the doctor has a hybrid role, she must conform to basic standards of professional ethics in relation to both the victim and suspect of crime, but she also has a clear duty arising from her policing responsibilities to law enforcement and public protection.

Similar questions can be asked about doctors and nurses in the armed services. The case of triage is well known, where often the highest levels of clinical need must go unmet in order to preserve the greatest chance of overall military effectiveness, And, of course, within the triage situation it is thus unreasonable to expect health professionals to discriminate purely on clinical criteria. Not all men and women will stand an equal chance of being treated based upon their level of injury, rather there will be military reasons for favouring certain people because of their position in the command chain, or their strengths, skills, or functions. Here healthcare is a servant of some other imperative and system of values and is almost entirely colonized by it

---

[1] At the time of writing the UK Parliament is making this practice lawful as a way of preventing drivers 'abusing' health grounds for deferring the taking of blood samples and thereby also evading the possibility of incriminating themselves by refusing the testing of the sample.

There are many other similar cases. Sorell, for example, uses the case of doctors in professional sport. But in all of these cases the health professional has more than one master. There is the 'patient' (or, perhaps more accurately, the person who is the immediate subject of their attentions) and there is some institution or social system to which they also owe responsibility. Given this situation there will necessarily be instances where there are overt conflicts of interest between the relevant parties. But these conflicts of interest are not surface, occasional, or accidental features of the situation. They are not the 'balancing acts' that come up from time to time, also rightly labelled as conflicts of interest, about which all professionals have to be ready to deliberate. They are permanent features of these scenarios, they are conflicts of interest which are embodied in the frameworks within which these health professionals work.

Why have I used these rather unusual examples and not even more radical examples about health professionals working for the Mafia or conducting state-sponsored torture? I have done so because I am interested in considering the strains within and between conceptions of professional legitimacy. It is difficult to know where professional ethics ends and straightforward abuse of professional knowledge and authority begins, but I am only interested here in the tensions which occur within those limits. I would want to resist the suggestion that the cases I have included here necessarily collapse into the ones I have put beyond the limits. There is simply not just one 'correct' position in ethical space for health professionals. Health professionals, like everyone else, are caught up with, and differentially positioned in, complex fields of obligations, interests, and ideals. What it is right for them to do depends to a large extent on what their 'job' is. Of course there are the two further questions: first, can this specific kind of role be ethically justified? Second, is this role being practised according to appropriate ethical standards? These questions are both of fundamental importance and they should not be evaded by imagining that the variety of roles can be reduced to some largely abstract ideal type of professional–patient relationship.

As I have mentioned above I think it is more fruitful to see all roles as 'anomalous' or, to avoid absurdity, to see all health-professional roles as embodying their own forms of hybridity.[2] Rather than see the police doctor as deviant we can emphasize the continuities between her work and the work of her colleagues practising health promotion, they too have some regard to public protection and even to the requirements of the law. In addition, as we have seen, they also have obligations to their other patients, to their colleagues, to their own friends and family, to the institutions that employ them, to their profession, and to the wider society.

---

[2] Sorell (2001) makes this point in relation to welfare-state health professionals in particular, but as I go on to explore there are not any clear distinctions between health systems in this regard.

In what remains of this chapter I want to concentrate mainly on the question with which I began it: how does the increasing 'role extension' of health professionals into public-health agendas or other social agendas reconfigure professional ethics? This is the example of hybridity that I have identified as central to the theme of this book. But before turning more explicitly to these issues I want to zoom in a little on one of the key worries about the protection of professional ethics under changing conditions, the preservation of trust between clients and professionals.

Preserving Trust

What has been said so far reflects what I take to be two widely shared assumptions. First, that effective systems of health-professional activity and professional ethics depend upon a good level of 'client trust' in professionals (as well, obviously, other conditions). Second, that such trust depends on a belief that the professional attaches a high priority to the protection and service of the client's interests. The issues I have been rehearsing amount to saying either that professionals can have more than one client which pulls them in different directions and/or that client interests may have to be balanced against other interests. This means that there is a chance that trust will be eroded or undermined.

Once again we are dealing with generalities here and it is very difficult, at least without imaginative and sensitive empirical research, to assess in real terms what these worries might amount to with respect to different kinds of professional roles and practices. However, it is possible to note that the nature of trust needed to underpin professional traditions is far from a clear-cut matter. There are at least three different dimensions to trust (a) There must be a degree of confidence in professional competence; competence here includes the appropriate set of technical, practical, and interpersonal forms of expertise; (b) There must be the assumption that the professional is honest and that the considerations which underpin advice or action are explained or can be opened up; and (c) There must be a readiness, where necessary or where it is sought, to be able to 'place oneself in the hands' of the professional, either because of sickness or lack of competence or expertise. The degree to which each of these three things is called for varies, and the overall level of trust needed also varies, depending upon the extent to which the client is practically dependent upon the professional and the importance of the potential benefits and risks. In short we can call these three factors clinical confidence, transparency and patient-centred beneficence.

The debate about the possible erosion of client trust, including the sorts of examples I have been discussing in these two chapters, has increasing relevance as we work through these three factors. There is no reason to suppose that the recognition of the hybrid nature of health-professional roles should in itself undermine clinical confidence. The issue is not primarily about whether professionals have the right skills and expertise but about the ends to which they put their expertise. Hybridity does however raise questions about transparency. If health professionals have conflicting loyalties, or conflicting ends in mind how far do they, or should they, obscure this fact? Finally, if clients believe that professionals are motivated by many things other than their clients' own immediate well-being, things such as system goals or public-health targets, why should they rely on professionals to act on their behalf?

An assessment of the potential erosion of patient trust in the light of changes in health policy, and associated role changes, depends upon considering these different elements and how they combine. Much of the literature on professional change uses human-resource language such as 'role extension' and 'new skill mix'. Changes of this sort are, of course, relevant to levels of clinical confidence because clinical confidence does to some extent depend upon stable expectations and well-understood roles. However, the real problem begins when we ask what it is best to do to underpin levels of trust in the light of professional change. Prima facie transparency is the most important consideration. What matters is that patients should understand as much as possible about the conflicting demands, constraints, and norms that shape professional roles. If a professional can only prescribe from within a severely curtailed and cost-limited formulary this ought to be explained. To do so restores what is arguably the fundamental condition of trust—honesty—and also treats the patient with proper respect. Yet to the extent that the patient wishes to 'transfer' his independence and choice-making to the professional, perhaps because the patient is feeling weak or vulnerable, and because he sees this 'letting go' as part of the caring and healing relationship, it would seem strange to insist on high levels of transparency. To do so might be less than caring.

Up to a point it seems fairly easy to say what needs to be done to preserve trust. There are minimal standards of transparency and beneficence. But there are many grey areas here. What, for example, can and should Debbie do to preserve the trust of Bridget and John in the relationship they have with her? Is it best for her to simply rely on their historical expectations about her beneficent intentions, or should she be more open about the health-promotion targets and norms which are steering her work with them?

Reconfiguring Professional Ethics: Trends in Policy and Practice

Of course health-professional roles have always been socially constructed. It was with this idea that I began Chapter 7. The positions that different professionals occupy in ethical space, their background sets of obligations and ideals, have always been established by social processes which are beyond their individual control. What I am discussing in this part of the book is not the social construction of roles as a new phenomenon. Rather I am reflecting on a whole compound of changes which have increased our collective self-consciousness about these processes of construction and certain movements which, I am suggesting, also amount to an intensification of the levels and kind of control exercised over health professionals. Professional regulation is built into the traditions, institutions, and very idea of professionalism. However, the historical emphasis was on establishing side-constraints on professional activity. There have always been certain things which professionals have been prohibited or strongly discouraged from doing by laws, codes of ethics, or 'custom and practice'. But within that the traditional paradigm professions—medicine in the arena of healthcare— have stressed the need for a high level of professional autonomy and personal judgement. For very many reasons this emphasis has gradually shifted. Indeed, virtually all of the themes discussed in this book are closely related to this shift: a social climate which has favoured 'empowerment' and client accountability over paternalism; the growth in the systemization and openness of professional knowledge and the evidence base; the increasing urgency of, and recognition of the need for, cost constraints and the stewardship of human and other resources; the growth in the techniques of and ideology of managerialism; and the public prominence of health policy and public-health agendas. All of these things conspire to produce closer forms of professional control.

But these changes should not only be seen as matters of control. They also constitute a compound and diverse set of changes to the value field of healthcare. In the examples at the beginning of this chapter the doctor may be responding to institutional norms or public-health targets but she may also be showing a personal and professional commitment to these things. It is too easy to simply fudge together as evidence of a single change what can be very different issues: cost-containment, managerial mechanisms, and a population orientation. Yes, an orientation towards the whole population rather than simply individual patients does press home the importance of financial stewardship, and managerial mechanisms are frequently used for this purpose. But both a population orientation and management, separately and in combination, can relate to many other goals. What I hope to be indicating more generally is the whole compound of ways in which healthcare professional roles are necessarily embedded in social agendas. To some extent these embedded norms will reflect 'vested interests' of one kind or another: commercial interests, the 'tribal' interests of occupational groups, macro- and micro-political interests, etc. But they also reflect, more or less explicitly, sets of competing social goals or ideals. These might be the goals of the healthcare system as a whole, or the goals of public health or broader social goals such as equity or solidarity (these three are obviously not exclusive categories). To repeat, not all of this change can be dismissed as the power of 'vested interests'.

I cannot do justice here to the many ways in which social agendas, of competing kinds, are embedded in professional roles. But I can continue to draw out the underlying thread that I have concentrated on thus far, namely the tension between individual and population-oriented approaches to health goods. To explore this issue further we can contrast an ideal type market-model of health provision and an ideal type welfare-state model with an explicit requirement on the health service to tackle inequalities in health. (The former is perhaps realized in pockets in many countries most notably the USA, the latter corresponds quite closely to the formal policy position of the New Labour government in the UK in the first years of the twenty-first century). It may be tempting for some to see the former as a 'pure model' and the latter as a 'hybrid model', in the sense that the lines of responsibility and service are relatively plain in model 1 and more obviously mixed, even muddy, in model 2. If I present myself to a doctor working in model 2, I might quite reasonably worry that the attention and resources that are devoted to me are determined by system and societal goods rather than solely according to my own needs. This is the case even supposing that the health professionals working in model 2 are very sophisticated and thoroughly beneficent, i.e. they know that most health inequalities can only be tackled by non-health service policies, and they are not disposed to refuse treatments to people simply because they are better off financially or medically. However, they also see that at the margins they can ameliorate some inequalities in health experiences by targeting resources and effort to some 'harder to reach' settings and people, and that some relatively healthy and affluent people might do perfectly well with some suboptimal treatment from the health service from time to time. A patient transferring from model 1 to model 2 may well feel that the professionals in it are less responsive to their needs as individuals rather than statistics, that these professionals are slightly more interested in 'intervention' than in 'consultation'. In turn this may undermine their trust in the professionals they encounter.

However, whilst granting all of this, I would not want to accept the idea that model 1 is somehow 'pure' compared to the hybrid nature of model 2. In both systems health professionals must serve system goals as well as individual goals, it is merely that the system goals are different in the two cases. In both systems the decisions of the professionals have clear effects on people other than the patients in front of them, including effects on inequalities in health. It is just that in one case these effects are self-consciously and explicitly built into the ideology of the system, in the other case they fall into the wider social ideology. Model 1 also has built into it risks of potential 'distortions', patients may have their needs inflated to some degree if this secures the profitability of the enterprise; treatment choices might be influenced, again at the margins, by the profile of in-house expertise and concerns about market share. These risks could perfectly reasonably undermine trust in the existence of patient-centred responsiveness. There is simply no such thing as 'one master' professionalism.

Health professionals are inextricably bound up in societal and system relationships as well as in client relationships. They cannot pretend that the broader social relationships merely provide a background platform to support their 'real work' with patients. On the other hand not many health professionals can define their role solely around some social ends such as the public health. For very many of them the reverse is true. They are typically engaged in caring relationships with specific individuals or groups of patients. They have to be able to work with person-centred agendas and to exercise a degree of 'representative partiality' to 'their' patients. As I suggested at the close of the last chapter the balancing acts here, between forms of 'impersonal' and 'personal' goods, are relevant to all health professional roles. From the issues I have been rehearsing it seems that there are three important considerations in assessing the necessary balances for specific roles. First, each role has to be seen in the context of its contribution to an overall division of ethical labour including, for example, divisions between population-oriented and patient-oriented outlooks and health outcomes and process goods. Second, for any health-professional role there must be a reasonable degree of public transparency about the goals, orientation, and 'rules of the game' that attach to the role. Third, the way the roles and responsibilities are defined must be able to be made relatively transparent whilst maintaining public confidence in the values of the health system and patient trust in the responsive and beneficent nature of professional care.

This is asking for a lot. Even if these balancing acts can be achieved within a health polity it seems to me that they require a new level of reflexivity and honesty on the part of health policy-makers and health professionals, and new forms of responsibility and realism on the part of patients and citizens. I would argue that in the recent evolution of healthcare systems these balancing acts have been undertaken in a largely covert and unselfconscious fashion, in many ways they have been hidden from both professionals and patients. The increasing importance of systems of professional control, almost always linked in with the discourses of stewardship, have brought about new balances by default. These constraining pressures have coincided with increasing professional aspirations to use new technologies, practise better psychosocial care, achieve more prevention, and, in some places, reduce health inequalities. Each of these countervailing pressures produces role extension and perhaps 'role stretch' for professionals who between them are in a position to do more for the individual patient and more for the population as a whole. The debates about resource allocation have developed as a response to these tensions and they provide a crucial ingredient for coping with them. However, debates about resource allocation should not be conducted in isolation from broader questions, not only the questions about the goals of the health system under consideration, which are implicit in them; but also questions about the changing nature of health-professional roles and ethics.

The value fields of healthcare create (and are created by) the ethical division of labour and the corresponding rules of the game: the obligation-sets, ideals, models of professionalism, and philosophies of health embodied in specific roles and in institutions. Any specific encounter in a healthcare setting takes place in a field with a particular profile of implicit values, e.g. particular balances between: treatment and prevention; cure and care; negative and positive conceptions of health; personal and impersonal outlooks; person-centred and population-centredness; individualism and solidarity; efficiency and equality, etc. As I have attempted to illustrate throughout this part of the book much of what is done by health professionals is so to speak 'done' before they begin to act. Any serious professional ethics must appraise both what professionals do, individually and collectively, and what is done by them. Similarly it needs to be concerned not only with what counts as the ethical boundaries of professional action, with 'unprofessional conduct', but also with the proper boundaries of professional roles.

PART 4

Education, Ethics, and Agenda-Setting

10

Rethinking Health Education

In this chapter I want to make a case for a new conception of health education which properly reflects a diffused health agenda, and diffused responsibility, and also to consider some of the dilemmas facing educators in this area. Discussions about all of the issues I have reviewed up to now are typically peppered with references to the importance of public education. I want to make the same point, that is, that there is a need for more and better public education about health-related matters. But I also wish to acknowledge two factors which are often neglected in these calls for education. First, it is quite common for 'education' to be cited as if it represented a comparatively unproblematic solution to some concern. (If group x were educated about y then problem z could be solved.) However, a little more reflection reminds us that questions about education are themselves both practically and ethically complex. Turning to education cannot be a way of evading health-policy problems; rather it is a way of opening up a further set of problems and contests. Second, there is a limit to how much 'education' alone, where this is understood as the 'inner learning' of individuals, can achieve unless it is embedded in changes in institutional and social relationships. For example, as I argued in Chapter 3, the relationships between health professionals and their clients have to be understood against the value fields, including the fields of power, which constitute them. Education, considered in isolation, is doomed to make little difference to presumptions of paternalism.

As a starting point I am happy to accept, and work with, Tones and Tilford's definition of health education:

Health education is any intentional activity that is designed to achieve health or illness related learning, i.e. some relatively permanent change in an individual's capability or disposition. Effective health education may, thus, produce changes in knowledge and understanding or ways of thinking; it may influence or clarify values; it may bring about some shift in belief or attitude; it may facilitate the acquisition of skills; it may even effect changes in behaviour. (Tones and Tilford, 2001: 301)

Tones calls this a 'technical definition' in order to signal his understanding that controversy ensues as soon as we begin to fill in the gaps in the definition, that is as soon as we ask about the purposes and content of health education (Tones, 2002: 1). It is precisely this, I think, which makes it a useful starting point. It is no more than a first unpacking of the conceptual pairing of health and education into a single phrase. It indicates the relative open-endedness of the idea of health education or, to put it slightly differently, the potential scope of the field of health education. Any activity aimed at any kind of health or illness-related learning is incorporated into this field.

This global conception of health education, which I will continue to rely upon, makes quite a sharp contrast with what I think are the most common and much narrower connotations of the expression 'health education'. These narrow connotations, it appears to me, link the notion of health education with strategies and techniques of medically led and instrumental public education. In short, health education is seen as the method by which necessary 'health messages' are transmitted to lay people. Assuming that I am right about this it raises a question about the reasons for this gap, and for the persistence of these narrow connotations in the light of the many and varied discussions about broader 'models' of health education in the health-education literature.

Health-Education Models

There are many different taxonomies of health-education models (Ewles and Simnett, 1995; Downie *et al.*, 1996; Tones and Tilford, 2001). These divide up the field of health education in different ways and according to different principles. Often they use slightly different names for essentially the same things. I will not try to capture all of this here. I am simply interested in illustrating the normative bases of health education and picking out those broad-value contests which are widely recognized and discussed. For these purposes I will use the best-known taxonomy which distinguishes between medical, educational, empowerment and social change models of health education.

The medical (or preventive) model of health education treats health education as a tool for disease management. Medicine has many tools for the management of disease and education is one of them. The point is that effective intervention is measured in relation to health outcomes. This means that the purposes and methods of intervention tend to be defined by medical agendas and expertise. Traditionally this model has been associated with trying to effect medically desirable patient-oriented behaviour change, whether 'lifestyle change' for preventive medicine or 'compliance' with medical treatment. As always there is an element of stereotyping and 'doctor bashing' in discussions about the medical model, but it is a useful ideal-type model if not taken too seriously as a description of doctors.

The educational model of health education is in many respects a reaction to the medical model. It stresses the importance of more open-ended means and ends. The point of health education, if it is to be education, is understanding and informed choice rather than specific health outcomes. Also, according to this model, health education should not be seen as a tool for bringing about attitude or behaviour change, rather it must use person-respecting methods which allow for greater equality and dialogue between 'teachers' and 'learners'. The educational model is perhaps most associated with the idea of informed choice, and for that reason is sometimes criticized for assuming high levels of individual freedom of action and not paying sufficient attention to the structural and cultural constraints faced by many people.

The empowerment model of health education addresses this concern about the obstacles to choice and action. It stresses the need for health education to take into account, and where possible develop, the internal and external resources which support health-related choices and action, and not only health-related understanding. Health educators who subscribe to this model aim to work with individuals in their communities to help them define and realize some of their goals. At a concrete level this might mean, for example, helping them set up a system of cycle lanes rather than just 'teaching them' about the value of cycling. As well as acknowledging the external environment of educational processes this model works with a more holistic model of education which recognizes the importance of embodied skills and confidence, etc. as well as abstract knowledge.

The social action (or radical) model of health education builds upon the notion of empowerment and in particular the need for structural change if the objectives of health education, in relation either to disease prevention or individual choice, are to be met. Sometimes 'top-down' change is stressed, e.g. government action on healthy public policies of various kinds; sometimes 'bottom-up' change is emphasized, e.g. self-help group or community politics, but health education from this perspective is linked to social and economic change and therefore must include a significant component of political education. Whatever else health education is about it must, according to this model, incorporate both an understanding of the social determinants of health and the development of political literacy. The empowerment and social action models, therefore, reflect the need, that I signalled above, for broader and more socially embedded approaches to education.

Of course this is only a sketch and these categories could be refined and combined in countless ways. But it is enough to show the contested nature of health education. This is, I think, the main benefit of the models debate. In some of the literature the models are referred to as if they represent a tool-box of 'approaches' to health education from which practitioners might pick and choose. But in reality they represent different value positions. The ideal-type models indicate different conceptions of legitimate means and ends. This distinction between means and ends is clearly important but, again, it is frequently lost in discussions of these ideal types which fudge them together. For example, the medical model is taken to suggest both 'disease-related outcomes' and 'expert-dominated persuasive tactics', when these things can, of course, exist separately from one another, and certainly need to be evaluated separately. From an evaluative perspective we must first distinguish between the different possible ends of health education, e.g. health outcomes, understanding, personal or community autonomy, or socio-economic change, and then, in general terms, and for specific settings and agents, consider the acceptability or merits of different pedagogies and curricula or educational content in conjunction with these ends.

There are a number of more theoretically informed discussions of health-education models (see Caplan and Holland, 1990; Beattie, 1991) which, amongst other things, draw out some of the underlying tensions inherent in the models debate. Simplifying these somewhat I will say that two main tensions are highlighted—the tension between an individualist or structural focus on the one hand, and between an 'authoritative' or 'negotiated' educational interaction on the other. These are sometimes represented as two intersecting axes which provide a two-dimensional map of possible health-education positions. (More precisely speaking a number of such maps have been produced with different axes but I will stick to this simple one here.) There is no necessary presumption, on my part or in the wider literature, that some positions are intrinsically better or worse than others. We need to look at the objectives, setting, and relationships involved in some detail to inform any such evaluation. Some circumstances may suggest the need for individually focused and authoritative educational interventions, perhaps, for example, 'persuading' infective TB patients of the reasons for, and importance of, taking their medication. I will return to some issues in the ethics of health education later, but this single example is enough to illustrate the close connection between the models debate and questions of ethics.

In the Name of Health Education

However, as I indicated at the start of this chapter, there is a substantial disjunction between the elasticity suggested by the models debate and the set of things which are commonly done in the name of health education. The former is fairly open-ended and the latter is fairly narrow. To make this claim definitively would require a systematic empirical investigation of the range of practices commonly described as health education. But I suggest that some reflection on our own experiences with, and intuitions about, real examples of health education will make this claim seem plausible. The expression 'health education' is often used in connection with 'bite-sized' messages such as 'Don't Drink and Drive', 'Eat five portions of fruit and vegetables a day', and 'Just say no to drugs'. In these cases we are dealing with simple imperatives, proscriptions and prescriptions which instruct individuals on the road to health improvement. Although these are extreme examples they capture something about a lot of health-education work. There are many posters, leaflets, and media campaigns which are principally designed around health-improvement messages. Very often these messages are set against the background of a more or less extensive information base, but normally this information is selected and presented with the rationale of supporting individuals to take steps to improve their own health. I suggest that it is these kinds of examples which are most typically conjured up by the idea of health education and that they are, in fact, broadly representative of the real-world 'flavour' of much health education. This is not surprising, nor would I suggest is it altogether a bad thing.

Health education has strong historical associations with medically led public-education work. (The education of professionals is separated off as, for example, 'medical education', 'nursing education', or is divided into academic domains such as 'health psychology', 'health economics', or 'health policy'.) This means that health education has existed most often as a technology of patient or public-health improvement, and should be understood in that light. It is only in that context that 'bite-size' messages can even be described as education without absurdity. (Imagine other educators confining themselves to similar slogans.) Historically health education has been 'education' for health and not education about health. Hence the huge gap between the definition I have adopted—'any intentional activity that is designed to achieve health or illness related learning'—and the narrow connotations of the term. In what follows I want to argue for a much broader and much more ambitious conception of health education.

To start with I would argue that the models debate is itself, in a number of respects, too narrow in scope. Partly this is because as well as including the medical model as just one component, the debate is in practice very often framed by the medical model. Health-education practitioners who are excited about the prospect of educational, empowerment, or social-action- style working find themselves in situations where the goals and parameters are medically defined. The job is, for example, to reduce heart disease by 5 per cent and the question is about what educational approach is best suited to achieve this objective. Within this framework all health education, however idealistic or holistic its self-perception, becomes instrumentalized and medicalized. This is not only a problem for practitioners constrained by policy demands. My reading suggests that exactly the same tendencies can often be seen in the theoretical debates about models.[1] The empowerment and social-action models are often discussed as if they were simply more effective methods of health promotion, and the educational model, which in many respects defines itself against the medical model, is very often partly assimilated to it. In many places the underlying assumption seems to be that education is for informed choice, because informed choice is the most effective medium of health promotion and not because it is viewed as a worthwhile end in itself.

But I do not want to claim much originality for these remarks. Critical currents in health education, both from philosophy and sociology, have pointed up this assimilation of health education to health promotion. They have illustrated the ways in which institutional settings and the discourses of biomedicine construct health education into an adjunct of medicine (and wider processes of social control). As part of this task they have drawn attention to the problem of defining 'ends' in health education, and in particular the need to place health-improvement ends in the context of other possible ends. However, I would want to add two other dimensions to this critique, dimensions which, I think, are rarely addressed in this context.

First, in rethinking health education we need to ask, 'who are the teachers and who are the learners?' The assimilation of health education to medicine is made easier by the parallels between doctor–patient and teacher–learner relationships. The presumption is that in matters of health the health professionals are the tutors and the public are the tutored. Of course this makes sense up to a point. In so far as we are talking about biomedical expertise about the prevention or treatment of disease it is important to acknowledge where the expertise lies. But the locus of expertise on very many other matters is much less easily discerned. This is increasingly acknowledged in developments such as the 'patient-expert' role and the representation of patient organizations in health regulation. However, there is still much more scope to press this question about the locus of expertise in health education.

Second, even assuming that we are talking about health education targeted at the general public, we can, and I think must, ask for a radically revised notion of what would count as relevant educational aims and content. There seems to be, in principle, no obvious limit to the kinds of themes, issues, and concerns that are worthy of serious public education work. For a start anything which is found in the curricula of health professionals, including the health-related academic domains within the social sciences and the humanities, must be of potential relevance; as must the policy issues that professionals and others grapple with in managing and delivering health

---

[1] Here I am going to simply assert this rather than give chapter and verse.

systems. All of these things and more could be done in the name of health education.

Education for a Diffused Health Agenda

The nature and role of health-related education has to adapt to the diffused health agenda. The diffused health agenda produces a changed education agenda, but also, and more fundamentally, the deeper historical and social currents which have affected healthcare also affect education in analogous ways. The diffused health agenda includes a greater understanding of the full set of health determinants, an enhanced emphasis on psychosocial dimensions of health experiences, and on broader conceptions of health, a concern with the distribution of health and ill-health and equity, and linked to all of these is the diffusion of responsibility for health. These trends all have both indirect and direct implications for education. Underpinning these trends, however, is a broader compound of social change which also challenges traditional models of education; these include: increased scepticism about professional authority and 'official knowledges' (Apple, 1993); changed patterns of social deference with more presumption of shared participation in decision-making; revised modes of regulation in welfare-related services, with a shift away from bureau-professional control towards managerial control; and closely linked to all of these shifts the increasing recognition of diverse voices and plural identities in social policy and politics (Lewis, Gewirtz, and Clarke, 2000). In this context restricted conceptions of health education make little sense. However, there is the problem of conceiving what should replace them that can do justice both to new health agendas and to less paternalistic conceptions of both healthcare and education.

It is not appropriate to consider all of these issues here but I need to mention some of them in order to move on to, and focus on, the relevance of wider conceptions of health education for the social context of healthcare ethics. There is the question of who is responsible for health education. Linked to this the consideration of the structures, settings, and media through which education is conducted. And, finally, the three matters I have introduced above. What is the right range of aims for health education, and how can these be balanced together? What are defensible approaches for this era of reconceived health education? What should be the content of such education?

Just as is the case with health there are no clear boundaries between educational and non-educational domains and settings, and no clear lines of 'ownership' of education. Education is in the hands of a broad range of private, public, and voluntary organizations including the family and peer groups. I will just make a few remarks which relate to certain key social agents: (i) government responsibility (at least as regulator if not as provider) for public education including both the compulsory phase in the education of young people, and for government-sponsored health information and education policies; (ii) the education and communication strategies of health providers and healthcare professional organizations, and (iii) those responsible for the training and professional development of health professionals whether in universities or workplace settings. In the first instance these comments will amount to little more than a rather glib 'wish list', but I will then turn to some of the complications they raise.

I would want to argue that it should be an imperative for all of the above agents to substantially increase the general level of health-related literacy. This is not simply because of the potential health gains which might be derived from people understanding more about the determinants of good health, i.e. health education as a technology of health improvement. It is also because without the opportunity to understand issues of health policy, healthcare, and health promotion people are effectively excluded from participation in, and shared responsibility for, health policy, i.e. health education as political education. Working with both sets of ends means moving decisively away from a simple diet of 'health promotion slogans' (although not necessarily abandoning these things) to a much richer diet of educational aims and approaches, where there are no sharp boundaries between professional and lay educational opportunities. This is essential in a health system where the limitations of technical expertise are well understood and where the responsibility for health is necessarily diffused. Many of the major problems of health policy now fall largely outside traditional forms of professional expertise, e.g. the management of chronic illness, priority setting, the ethics of new reproductive technology.

If this more demanding educational agenda is not addressed in a determined way then, I would suggest, the fundamental underpinning of healthcare paternalism will be left in place. As I have indicated elsewhere healthcare paternalism is not intrinsically bad: whether or not paternalism is defensible depends upon the case in question. However, this also means that the presumption of paternalism must be questioned, and there must be the possibility of, and mechanisms for, greater power-sharing in healthcare. As things stand I would argue that the monopolizing of 'health policy and healthcare knowledge' by health professionals underscores a general presumption of paternalism in health. This has implications for every educational sector. Generally the shift must be from health education on a 'need to know basis' to health education on an equal basis.

In compulsory education for young people there is plenty of opportunity to begin to restore the balance. In these contexts education about health does not need to be separated from welfare or well-being related themes. The tradition of PSHE (personal, social, and health education in schools) provides a basis for future developments. But it is also important to ensure that (a) PSHE is not dominated by individual-centred lifestyle-related approaches but sets these in the context of political education; (b) that all of these PSHE themes are not insulated from other more formal, and more assessed, curriculum areas. In compulsory schooling the strong separation of 'practical' health-related topics and themes, from 'pure' academic domains works, in effect, as a device of professional exclusion. The full richness and complexity of the health-related subject domains is preserved for those entering the health professions. It is increasingly recognized that this serves neither academic nor practical agendas. Both are diminished by this separation of practical relevance and disciplinary frameworks. For example, there are now strong calls from school science educators to ensure that there is sufficient attention to value questions and the social context of science within school science curricula (not to dissolve the discipline-centred approaches but to complement them) (Millar and Osborne, 1998). This requires rethinking curricula, teaching, and learning but the alternative is to reinforce the relative closure of many professional and policy domains.

Government-sponsored health information and health education should be organized around a very different philosophy. Too often, at present, the emphasis is upon nuggets of health information rather than on education for participation. This is made manifest by the policy of focusing predominantly on 'tip of the iceberg' issues. Where there is a major matter of public concern, the government provides information and 'reassurance' to counter that concern. This, for example, was the approach taken during a recent UK concern about the safety of the combined Measles, Mumps, and Rubella (MMR) vaccine. The media stories and public discussion surrounding this concern provided an excellent opportunity for wider public education about the nature of epidemiological knowledge and scientific uncertainty which was almost entirely missed. In this context the official medical authorities and 'worried' lay representatives seem to play the same anti-educational game. The latter complain about the lack of complete reassurance and 'certainty', and the former offer as much reassurance and 'certainty' as they feel able to muster, rather than sharing the extent of, and reasons for, uncertainty and the rationale for their policy line. In doing this public-health agents operate in an analogous way to clinicians of 25 or more years ago when there was a greater presumption of the benefits of paternalism. I will come back to some of the ethical issues raised here later in the chapter, but broadly speaking I want to suggest that respect for, and involvement of, 'health consumers' cannot be confined to the microcontexts of healthcare.

Although there is a limit to the extent to which healthcare providers and health-professional organizations can be charged with a general public education remit I would argue that the same principles apply to them. As well as having specific duties for providing person-specific information to the individuals with whom they deal, they have some allied duties to provide education about the policies and practices which provide the context for individual decision-making. At a minimum, for example, a large hospital cannot regard itself as fully meeting its duties of accountability if it does not at least provide the opportunity for the community which it serves to learn about its priorities and procedures and the reasoning which informs them. Similarly a professional body should not be advising its members about 'good practice' in relation to specific issues without that information, and the evidence base and arguments which underpin the advice, at least being widely disseminated. More ideally such advice should spring from a climate in which both professionals and patient representatives are reviewing practice in the public gaze. Individual health professionals have analogous responsibilities, to play their part in these general education processes, in their relationships with patients and the wider community.

Those responsible for the education of health professionals, for example, in medical schools, nursing schools, or in professional placements, must consider how the organization and content of this education serves to 'separate out' professionals and the public. To some extent professional education is, by definition, about professional separation and there is a limit as to how far it is an intelligible aspiration to avoid separation. However, it seems to me that the traditional patterns of professional education are clearly excessive in this regard. In an era with a diffused health agenda, with the social context seen as central to healthcare, with lay conceptions of health taken seriously, and with the responsibility for health itself diffused, lay perspectives need to be properly incorporated into professional education. This means both (a) ensuring that lay perspectives and allied ideas about partnership and participation in healthcare and health policy are taught about, and experienced, in professional programmes, but also (b) that non-specialist and non-professional voices are given a serious part to play both in the organization of, and the delivery of, such programmes. This need not mean abandoning the considerable freedom of health-professional groups to determine their own education pathways, but rather should mean balancing that freedom a little more with other considerations.

In short what I am arguing for is a far greater emphasis upon education, understood broadly, as both a means and an end of health policy and health-professional activity. Educational goods ought to be a well-recognized subset of health goods, and more substantially embedded in the value field of health-related action.

Dilemmas in Reforming Health Education

But, as I have noted, these ideas and aspirations are somewhat glib. They are provided as a sketch of some very general concerns and possible directions with, as yet, very little consideration as to their practicability or defensibility. In this section I want to consider some potential problems with rethinking health education along these lines, with particular reference to the ethical issues it raises. To do so I need to return to some of the tensions and dilemmas embedded in the models debate.

The fundamental tension I have identified is that between health education as a technology of health improvement and health education as political education. These notions are only idealizations but each of them, and the tensions between them, indicate the relevant field of ethical concerns. Health education as a health-improvement technology emphasizes public-health outcomes, medical paternalism, and the dissemination of 'need to know' health information. Health education as political education emphasizes understanding for participation, client, consumer, or public autonomy, and the opening up of 'expertise'. My suggestions have stressed the importance of the latter in its own right and as a necessary feature of diffused health agendas. However, it is important neither to ignore the potential value of health-improvement models, nor to neglect the potential harm or wrong that might be caused by undue emphasis on health-related political education.

The tensions represented here are those which run through many of the discussions in this book, and much more importantly are at the heart of all modern healthcare and health-policy debates. How far can and should health policy treat individuals as sites for technical intervention, as 'objects' which can be manipulated for the beneficent management of health and disease? Or how far ought health policy to be constructed more collectively, through, for example, professional and 'patient' partnerships, in which individuals are treated as equal 'thinking subjects' and healthcare agents? As I indicated earlier in the chapter the tendency to date has been for health education to be conceived according to the former picture, as simply one further technology analogous to water purification or vaccination. These two pictures push in very different directions. In the former case the question to be asked is only 'what works'. Rather than ask what individuals might (in any sense) benefit from knowing about and understanding, or what they are entitled to know, we ask 'What information, in what form, is effective for health improvement?' A review of health-education journals will uncover countless 'scientific papers' analysing health-education initiatives in precisely these terms. An education 'purist' may well be inclined to say that this line of reasoning is simply not education at all but something more like coercion or manipulation. To some extent the concerns of 'health' and 'education' might well come into conflict here. Health outcomes have not come to prominence simply because of the dominance of biomedical discourse, they also, normally at least, represent inherently valuable ends. And if some health can be 'bought' at the expense of an educational compromise might that not be a reasonable price to pay?

It is worth briefly looking at some examples. Breast-screening programmes are typically well considered, carefully researched, and professionally organized health services. One important consideration facing those responsible for breast-screening programmes is how to strike the right balance in the kinds and levels of information dissemination and education which support such programmes. Information has to be designed to ensure that women attend and understand something about the purpose of the screening, the possible pain or discomfort involved, and the potential consequences of screening (for example, the possibility of being invited back for further tests). It makes sense for those responsible for the programme to undertake, or review, trials about the impact of different approaches to invitation or information on the overall effectiveness of the programme, as indicated by factors such as levels of uptake and user satisfaction. It would be odd, indeed arguably irresponsible, if information and education strategies were not informed by these kinds of studies and considerations. Set against this it also makes good sense, however, to ask what the women who are directly or indirectly affected by the existence of a programme *ought* to know about it. For example, how much ought they to know about things like false positives and false negatives, the possibilities for treatment, should this prove necessary, post-screening, or even about expert disputes about the potential side effects of screening or its overall effectiveness? (Dines, 1997). Here there seems to be a need for access to different kinds of information and for more or less superficial or in-depth sorts of health education. It would not make sense for the information accompanying routine invitations to screening to be accompanied by substantial digests of epidemiological and cost-effectiveness studies. On the other hand these rich sources of evidence and analysis are in the public domain, and health services and professionals need to decide if and how to support members of the public who want help accessing them or interpreting them.

This example does more than just illustrate the tension between 'education for health outcomes' and 'education for participation'. The emotional sensitivity of this field highlights another important dimension of technological and paternalistic approaches to health education: the importance of psychological protection. This is most obvious in relation to the communication of diagnoses in clinical settings. Assuming that people have a clear entitlement to know what is wrong with them and what the implications of diagnoses are, it does not follow that they need to be 'instructed' in detail and in full about these things on day one. If a medical consultant discovers a significant abnormality in heart function, it does not follow that he or she is then and there obliged to explain possible illness trajectories and the likelihood of serious illness and death. In many cases we would no doubt judge this level of immediate disclosure to be irresponsible conduct. Individuals obviously need time, space, and support to take things on board. The detached and 'matter of fact' attitudes that are often appropriate to the 'outside' professional perspective are usually not available from the 'inside' patient perspective. Here patient information and education has to proceed at a pace that is compatible with, and in careful balance with, patient protection in a way that is responsive to the needs and demands of particular patients. This need to protect people from threatening health information is understandably built into health-professional cultures. To some extent this culture affects all forms of health education whether or not it should. Breast-cancer screening is an intermediate case where the people being communicated with are directly affected by the service, and may be so in ways that touch them deeply. Educational initiatives which are designed as part of the screening programme, therefore, have to consider what may be the conflicting demands of health promotion, understanding, and psychological protection. Within this specific context there is arguably little case for open-ended education for education's sake.

The same seems to apply to the MMR triple-vaccine example mentioned earlier. The vaccination service itself cannot be in the business of open-ended education. It is dealing directly with concerned, and often anxious, parents whose attention is powerfully focused upon the welfare of their children. As a result it also has to think carefully about how it constructs invitations and information about the vaccine, and how it answers questions bearing in mind both the likely effects on health outcomes and the potential effects on parental confusion and distress. Again, the different ends (health, understanding, and peace of mind) which sometimes pull in opposite directions have to be balanced together.

However, I would suggest that these examples merely confirm the need for much broader and deeper health-education agendas. They show that there are limits to, and balancing acts within, some specific health-service-related communication strategies. In particular there is a case to be made sometimes for 'simpler' action-oriented messages and for 'reassurance'. However, the existence of these kinds of strategies merely underscores the need for a set of complementary and more open, complex, and problematizing forms of health education. Unless we assume that all health-related discourses are to be framed by professional paternalism and public protection, and that health education is only going to operate with useful simplifications and myths, there must also be spaces and possibilities for open-ended and exploratory education about health policies, including health education about the challenges of health education. These examples also point to the need for health education to operate in spaces outside those where people are immediately affected as 'insiders'. If health-related education is only to take place when there is a premium on 'care' and psychological protection it will always be circumscribed by non-educational concerns. Hence my proposals, sketched in the previous section, for much more extensive models of health education. There must be arenas in which the uncertainties surrounding such things as breast-cancer screening or vaccination can be shared and collectively considered and debated if the notion of public-health education is to be meaningful.

Thus re-envisaging health education along the lines I have suggested gives rise to practical and ethical dilemmas. There is no panacea of 'perfect' health education. All packages of health education will be contentious. But, as I am also suggesting, part of the way forward is to make these kinds of dilemma part of the content of health education. This cannot be done by the use of discrete educational initiatives let alone simple messages (the notion of specific educational interventions is itself a product of 'medical-model' thinking) but requires a large-scale and holistic conception of health-related education. 'Health' understood variously as 'absence of disease', 'welfare', and 'well-being' is a very major concern for individuals and for society as a whole. If education has a role either in helping people understand and change their physical and cultural environment, or in helping them to learn how to live their own lives and in communities, then health education (in the global sense) should have a central role in all sectors and settings. As I argued earlier health is one of the few 'goods' which is held in common in these times of cultural and value pluralism. Of course in practice one of the first jobs of health education will be to problematize this idea of health as 'one good' and open up the range and contestedness of 'health goods', but nonetheless health represents a fundamentally important meeting point for many forms of education.

Compulsion and Choice

The 'new' health education that I am advocating acknowledges the place of education as a healthcare technology but is closer to the ideal type of health education as political education. As well as arguing for much more health education I am arguing that it is necessary to increasingly play up those ends which are broader than the production of 'health outcomes', ends such as understanding, healthcare participation, and most generally citizenship. One important part of this new educational agenda is the dissemination of health-policy dilemmas of all kinds, for example, dilemmas about resource allocation, the role of the state in healthcare provision, regulation of and access to pharmaceuticals, the use of new technologies (assisted reproduction, genetic, etc.), the health inequalities agenda, and so on. If there is to be any prospect of wider 'democratic deliberation' about these issues of health policy including health-policy ethics this cannot be left to one-off processes of public consultation but rather requires a climate in which people have opportunities to familiarize themselves with these kinds of issues and can practise thinking and talking about them. Of course not everyone will have the inclination to involve themselves in this way, and arguably some people may lack the capacity, but, as I want to discuss now, this latter should not simply be presumed.

At base the difference between the 'healthcare technology' and the 'polit-ical-education' models is that the former treats people as objects and the latter treats people as subjects. In the technological approach what matters is technical control of behaviour. Cultural norms, subjectivities, or states of mind are treated as media for public-health change in just the same way as the air or water supplies are. What matters is using the causal mechanisms which will bring about the desired health outcomes. This may require 'inter-vention' to change norms or intentions, and the technical effectiveness of these interventions is what determines their worth. (If anyone doubts the practical relevance of these remarks they need to acquaint themselves with the health-promotion sciences literature.) From this perspective there is no important distinction between 'persuasion' and education. If we are putting together an advertising campaign to discourage people from taking illegal drugs, we will think first and foremost about what might produce that effect, and we will plan our market research on that basis. The result may include shocking images or much more subtle forms of symbolism designed to work through subconscious or unconscious processes. This approach is exempli-fied by what has been called the 'social marketing' approach to health education, the adoption by health educators of the attitudes and techniques of marketing for 'pro-social' ends.

From an educational point of view the problem, of course, is that market-ing has only an external relation to truth. Those who are 'marketing' health may be concerned that they are not 'selling' falsehoods but once they have reassured themselves on that score they do not need to be concerned about communicating the bases of truth claims nor about opening up truth claims for critical examination. Thus, in the example we are considering here, the marketers may well satisfy themselves that the 'message' about drug harms is accurate but it is not part of their remit to make the reasoning behind this conclusion explicit, nor to present some alternative and conflicting accounts of drug use which they have chosen to discount. The adverts that result therefore amount to little more than well-intentioned manipulation. This is precisely what so much clinical healthcare ethics has been pushing against for the past 25 years. A more educational approach to this topic would be completely different. Here I am thinking of what I have previously called 'education for understanding', or even the strongly normative conception of education defended by R.S. Peters (1966) in which 'education', to earn the title, must aim at worthwhile ends, use person-respecting methods, and involve a 'wide cognitive perspective'. Education, so understood, has an internal relation to truth and truth claims. The processes of education cannot simply convey ideas but must explore and analyse competing sets of ideas in context, their foundations and implications, and do so in partnerships between teachers and learners.

Social organization no doubt requires both persuasion and education. It is, I suggest, naïve to suppose that systems of incentives and disincentives, and forms of social policing and regulation, could be wholly replaced by educational approaches. There is no reason to suppose that this is a sensible proposition; quite the opposite. We know, I suggest, from our own cases that we are not always motivated by our 'educated insights' but often by more immediate and more basic intuitions and instincts; and the latter need to be sometimes harnessed for collective ends. However, it is perfectly meaningful and sensible to ask about the possible balances between persuasion and education, and where these might be and ought to be different. It seems to me that persuasion and manipulation for the public good may well be defensible in specific cases, but it is much more easily defended if there are proper educational opportunities for people to understand and participate in its defence. For example, road-safety campaigns which encourage safer driving in combination with various kinds of road design and traffic regulation may be founded on manipulative tactics. They may work because of the creation of 'optical illusions' or the appeal to primitive fears. To this extent they are treating the road-users as objects to be manipulated. The users here are not treated in an essentially different way than the cars. Assuming that the decision-making behind this is publicly accountable in some way I would want to argue that there is nothing intrinsically wrong with this treatment. But I cannot see how the requirements of public accountability can be properly met unless there are also complementary educational processes aimed at building wider literacy about road-safety policies and the strategies and dilemmas built into them.

There is a fundamental ethical difference between health policies being realized through persuasion and manipulation or through participation; the less people are compelled to 'comply' with the requirements of the public good and the more they choose to act on the basis of an understanding of the public good the better. (As I have been arguing in practice this may sometimes be the difference between being 'compelled' with more or less consent.) This is true for a number of reasons. First, the exercise of autonomy is a good; autonomy is a good thing in itself, it is a key component of what enables people to live a life that is worth living. Second, the more genuinely consensual policies are the lower the practical and ethical 'costs' of social-control mechanisms. Third, there are real limits to what can be achieved through social-control mechanisms and without the substantial resource of diffused intelligence and agency, especially in complex matters. Consider, for example, an approach to the HIV/AIDS epidemic which did not seek to recruit and involve individuals as informed and responsible citizens but concentrated solely on a combination of social marketing and policing tactics. Here, and in many other instances, it seems that the addition of the former, more inclusive, approach is likely to be not only much more respectful but also much more effective.

Healthcare Ethics and Education

In Chapter 4 I drew attention to the need for healthcare ethics to consider all of the 'forms of influence' which operate in healthcare and health policy including educational influences. I have begun to consider some of the relevant issues in this chapter, and I will not attempt to explore the ethics of health education in any more depth here. Rather I will conclude the chapter by making a few provisional comments about a rather different question: within my re-imagined health education what is the potential place of healthcare ethics?

Education for a diffused health agenda is education for diffused responsibility, and, therefore, is necessarily both political education and moral education. The health-policy debates and dilemmas discussed in this book, and briefly listed earlier in this chapter, are often substantially more complex than the health-promotion technology examples (drugs and road-safety campaigns) considered in the previous section. They frequently involve multilayered compounds of dilemmas in health-policy ethics. A debate about the regulation of assisted reproduction, for example, may well raise questions about the status of embryos, women's rights, ageism, resource allocation, the scope of public-service provision, family policy, and many other things. Each of these elements is highly contested and when they are compounded into what are frequently socially and emotionally contentious 'topics' they are extremely difficult to analyse coolly and carefully. This is the task that philosophically informed healthcare ethics has taken upon itself, and in so doing healthcare ethicists are typically (and quite reasonably) keen to distinguish their approach from that often pursued by portions of the media or vested-interest groups. Healthcare ethics as a discipline strives for a measure of detachment and balance and for the public audit of lines of reasoning. This is typically—and, again, I think rightly—contrasted favourably with the parading of 'gut feelings' and prejudices deployed by less responsible pundits. I say 'rightly' because what lies behind it is precisely the same concern with truth and the status of truth claims that elevates education above manipulation.

Healthcare ethics as a discipline is, in one sense, entirely accessible to members of the public. There is no particular barrier to stop anyone reading texts, attending conferences, undertaking courses in the field. Furthermore a number of senior healthcare ethicists put time and effort into communicating their work through popular media. However, I suggest that more can and should be done to disseminate the work, and the approaches, of healthcare ethics across society more generally. There is plenty of scope for work on these themes in schools, in further and higher education, and in popular fora. It seems to me essential that healthcare ethicists do not fall into some of the same 'distancing' traps that have plagued other forms of health-professional expertise. Obviously there is a limit to the extent to which people in general will be inclined to take an interest, and to the amount they are ready and able to learn from what may sometimes be 'watered down' treatments of the issues. Nonetheless there is a lot to be gained by creating a climate in which engagement with the themes and topics of healthcare ethics is relatively routine rather than occasional and ad hoc. There is precisely the same need for more widespread 'value literacy' as there is for more widespread scientific literacy, indeed these things often need to go together. Healthcare ethics, like science, should be high on the priorities of those with an interest in public education.

This call for broader education about, and involvement in, policy dilemmas does not rest upon the simplistic assumption that 'more heads are always better'. In many cases we have good reasons to suppose that mass decision-making will be worse than focused decision-making. As I argued in Chapter 3 democratic involvement cannot be a substitute for the rigorous application of independent standards by properly informed and authorized agents. But broader involvement is important if: (a) we are to treat everyone with respect and allow for the possibility that any contribution may turn out to be a valuable one; (b) we want to ensure that policy decisions are open to public scrutiny, and (c) we wish to gain as much as possible from good-quality processes of democratic deliberation both as ends in themselves, and as epistemological devices for learning from diverse perspectives and agents.

Health education, in the narrow forms in which it has predominated, has frequently been seen as a Cinderella educational field. Rather than being 'proper education' it has too often been a mechanism of social regulation using its target audience as instruments for public-health objectives. Here I have been trying to stress the potential of health education as a genuinely educational field. But one thing about the existing tradition of health education is to be admired; that is, it has often been directly geared towards action and towards valuable ends. What is needed, I have claimed, is not only an education for understanding but also an education for action which: (i) is based upon treating people as subjects not just as objects, (ii) is based upon broader and more self-consciously debated notions of what might count as valuable ends, and (iii) is closely linked to genuine mechanisms of inclusion in health-related decision-making. If we are to share responsibility for health we need more than an intellectual understanding of things like health determinants and health-policy dilemmas. Political education must also encompass 'moral education' in the traditional sense in which it is concerned with the cultivation of the virtues necessary to practise effective citizenship. Overall we need to foster a strong sense of how we are personally and collectively positioned with regard to these determinants and dilemmas, and the inclination and courage to make a contribution to addressing them.

11

Towards a Socially Reflexive Healthcare Ethics

In these two concluding chapters I want to pull together the arguments and implications of the book. In particular I want to ask about how we, individually and collectively, ought to understand and debate the major questions of public-health policy. In doing so I will also return explicitly to the idea of setting healthcare ethics in social context and to the two themes with which I opened the preface, the social construction of health goods and health as a social good. Although, as I have argued elsewhere, the methodological and substantive themes of the book are strongly interrelated, I will concentrate in this chapter upon the methodological implications of my arguments, i.e. the implications of my arguments for the direction of healthcare ethics. In the final chapter I will put more emphasis upon the substantive implications, i.e. the implications for the direction of the health agenda.

Healthcare Ethics as Public-Health Ethics

One way of summarizing both my methodological and substantive arguments is to stress that public health is central to healthcare ethics. I am arguing that as well as seeing 'public-health ethics' as a branch of healthcare ethics we should see it as an ingredient of all healthcare ethics. In the first case we have in mind the ethical appraisal of certain kinds of health-related intervention, those specifically aimed at population health. In the second case, I am suggesting, we should have in mind: (a) the ways in which all healthcare both shapes, and is shaped by, broader social and public-policy agendas, and (b) that, therefore, the ethical appraisal of any aspect of healthcare needs to be sensitive to and informed by these broader agendas.

As I argued in Chapter 4 to label an issue as an issue in 'healthcare ethics' (whether, in relation to clinical ethics or public-health ethics) is a product of our 'framing' practices. This framing happens both at a purely conceptual level and because our discourses are embodied in social and institutional frameworks. Through these framing practices we construct, and thereby to some extent 'separate off', a realm of healthcare from other dimensions of the social field. What I have called the diffusion of the health agenda brings about an ever-wider recognition of the difficulties of any such separation. On the one hand, for example, there is the seemingly endless potential for more and better-health promotion. On the other hand there is the corresponding concern about the ever-more intrusive 'medicalization' of our lives. These kinds of trends make us more aware of, and more reflexive about, the blurred boundaries between healthcare and the rest of life, and this makes stronger kinds of framing with regard to healthcare and healthcare ethics less plausible. Moving our attention away from the relatively well-defined frame of the one-to-one clinical encounter and in the direction of more diffused interventions also highlights a number of ethically important practical and philosophical debates (which are ever-present but not always equally prominent): (i) debates about the ends of health-related interventions; (ii) debates about knowledge or expertise; (iii) debates about legitimacy or authorization; (iv) debates about the relevant locus of agency and responsibility; and (v) debates about the distribution of health and health opportunities.[1]

In the remainder of this section I want to summarize what I think this 'opening out' of the ethical agenda adds up to for the focus and methods of healthcare ethics by: (a) reviewing their implications for a 'revised' public-health ethics, and (b) further elucidating what I mean by saying that such a public-health ethics should be an ingredient of all healthcare ethics.

Appraising childhood vaccination schemes. For illustrative purposes I will use a classic public-health dilemma, namely the provision and 'policing' of childhood vaccination schemes, i.e. how far is it ethically defensible to use different forms of 'social influence' (exhortation, dis/incentives, compulsion, etc.) to ensure that individuals comply with vaccination policies that are designed to serve the good of a population? Looked at in the narrowest of terms this dilemma rests upon two core concerns: (i) judgements about the health benefits and risks of a particular vaccination scheme and (ii) some reading of the right 'balance' between respecting individual choice on the one hand and improved public health on the other. Following from the arguments I have rehearsed above (and, I should stress, from arguments also reflected in other recent currents of work in bioethics) I would want to see these core concerns

---

[1] In the case of more diffused interventions these philosophical and practical debates become conspicuous and, once highlighted, these factors add extra layers of uncertainty to the inherently dilemmatic nature of healthcare ethics. Hence in the case of examples such as national policies promoting 'safe sex' or 'healthy drinking' the complications rehearsed here are evident, whereas in the case of examples such as a clinician negotiating a treatment some of these complicating factors are 'framed out' either (a) because they have less relevance or (b) because their relevance is 'put on one side'. I am arguing that we need to interrogate the balance between (a) and (b), otherwise it is not clear when we have satisfied ourselves that ethically relevant considerations have been considered and when we are simply overlooking them.

complemented by, or interpreted through, a range of other and overlapping concerns including questions about: (a) *broader policy ends and effects* in relation, for example, to education or 'community development'; (b) the *different kinds of knowledge* and forms of reasoning that are relevant to judging the practices inherent in, and the various effects of, such schemes; for example the potential role of interpretative as well as more positivist kinds of social inquiry; and (c) the *macro- and micro-contexts* under scrutiny, that is, for example, what are the background assumptions of the health polity in question and exactly what happens in the transactions between those administering a scheme and the individuals affected by it? In a moment I will expand on each of these concerns in turn and in so doing try to draw out their interrelationships with one another and with what I labelled the core concerns above.

The account I am offering here is merely a variant of a familiar story. The two core concerns set out above can be construed, and approached, as in the first case a technical–factual question about medical evidence which falls largely within the scope of epidemiological methods, and in the second case as an abstract puzzle for philosophical ethics about individual autonomy versus population utility. This division of labour between, and combination of, a broadly 'empirical' approach to medical facts and a broadly 'rationalist' approach to healthcare values is a legacy of positivist traditions whose influence lingers on despite pervasive and powerful critique. A number of the points I am making can be read as simply another version of this critique. I want to resist this particular division of academic labour and I want to do so not just because I see the empirical and ethical questions as strongly interwoven and interdependent but also because it seems to me that in practice this division often serves to mask the kinds of complementary concerns that I want to emphasize.

Broader policy ends and effects. Childhood vaccination schemes are, of course, aimed at reducing the incidence and prevalence of certain diseases and thereby the prevention of suffering and loss of life. This is their core purpose and it would be foolish to pretend that they are *really* designed for some other purpose. (For less classic public-health policies, such as the example of 'tackling teenage pregnancy' used earlier, this sort of worry is far from foolish.) However, it is certainly important to ask about both the 'secondary purposes' that such schemes might serve and also their 'side effects'. Furthermore, I would want to insist that the ethical defensibility of specific kinds of social influence on choice-making depends, amongst other things, on a full consideration of the potential purposes and effects of specific schemes. We cannot decide what practices are acceptable unless we are clear about what we are aiming to do, or practically doing, through these practices.

Let us assume that the vaccination scheme we are considering is very effective at reducing morbidity and mortality and therefore, even if it has significant health risks for a minority, has a compelling appeal from a utilitarian point of view. What other ends and effects might have relevance to its appraisal? Some other ends which vaccination schemes could serve (and which could therefore be taken into account in their design and defence) include: (a) general education about health, the causation of ill-health, and responsibilities for health protection and promotion; (b) education about or encouragement or enforcement of shared public-health obligations, and (c) the cultivation and reinforcement of a sense of civic identity and solidarity. The place of these kinds of purposes may at first sight seem relatively limited compared to the more obvious preventive functions of vaccination but I think that is probably a mistaken view. What is at stake here are very large questions about the relationships between, and the sharing of responsibilities between, those running health systems and those who are served by health systems. These are questions about the levels of paternalism and levels of involvement that underpin such systems, and about the degrees of 'owner- ship' and responsibility individuals are able and willing to take for the systems that support their health. Of course childhood vaccination schemes are only one relatively confined arena for determining and shaping these matters, and they need to be seen in the context of the system as a whole (see below). But those of us who attach weight to relational, educational, and participative goods as intrinsic to healthcare systems,[2] i.e. who see health and healthcare as about, in fundamental respects, shared goods and shared responsibilities, cannot sensibly appraise any public-health intervention without paying regard to these kinds of goods.

Having noted this broader perspective, however, it is also important to note that there are no straightforward moves linking the acknowledgement of these goods to the defensibility of vaccination schemes. Indeed, I would argue that, this broader perspective points us in two contrasting directions. On the one hand it provides an extra dimension of justification for using some stronger forms of social influence to make manifest and underpin our shared public-health obligations. On the other hand it reinforces the import- ance of informed and willing participation in such schemes, the necessary levels of understanding and willingness being in themselves constitutive of our collective identity and well-being.

Nonetheless it seems to me that, however confusing or complicating it is to bring into view aspects of this wider canvas, ethical appraisal can only be improved if we are sensitive to, and take into account, a proper range of

---

[2] At this stage in the book I will merely assume that I am right, for reasons set out earlier, about the importance of these factors. I will just note in passing that some people may want to argue for a more individualist/ 'privatized' conception of healthcare and healthcare responsibil- ities. Here I am simply not considering this alternative perspective.

relevant considerations. Suppose, for example, that we are asked to appraise a proposed policy—a policy which applies in certain states—that entry to schooling should be contingent upon evidence of having been administered specific vaccines. How should we proceed? As I have already said it seems that there will often be a strong utilitarian justification for such a policy. The population of schoolchildren, and the wider population, will only be adequately protected if sufficient numbers are vaccinated and, although the modelling of risks and benefits may show that there is little additional risk if a small minority of people avoid compliance, it is also arguable that: (a) the health of the majority cannot be entirely left to individual private-regarding choices, (b) that as a consequence individuals 'owe it to one another' to comply with such schemes, and (c) that for these reasons some degree of social coercion, in this instance using school entry as a mechanism, is justifiable. In the case of childhood vaccination there is also, of course, a plausible case for state paternalism aimed at the future health of people who are not themselves in a position to make informed choices and whose parents or caregivers may happen to be ill-informed or otherwise dislocated from preventive-medicine schemes, e.g. because of other demands on their attention or resources. These prima facie justifications would, it seems to me, be reinforced if the scheme is designed and works in a way that helps those who participate in it to appreciate both the overwhelming clinical rationale for using a population-oriented approach to infectious disease control and also the importance of the relational goods that can be embodied in such population-oriented health action.

But all of this is too abstract. What is needed to make any real progress with such an appraisal is a grounded understanding of what happens in, or more exactly what it is actually possible to achieve in, specific contexts. This is why we need to be sensitive not only to the full range of policy ends but also to the full range of policy effects. We need to be able to make well-grounded judgements about how far such schemes can and do serve educational functions, or build forms of solidarity, or how far they can and do have very different effects, for example, breeding resentment and producing resistance to, and alienation from, health systems, policy-makers, or health professionals. This takes me on to the other two complementary considerations I introduced above: the relevance of a variety of forms of knowledge and attention to contexts.

Different kinds of knowledge. In talking about the relevance of different kinds of knowledge I have in mind first and foremost a concern that I will return to later in this chapter and in the next, i.e. the need for healthcare ethics to be properly interdisciplinary, or in other words for it to decisively move away from an equation that defines healthcare ethics as medical knowledge plus law and philosophy. This interdisciplinary trend is now well underway although there is still a tendency for work in the field to be merely multidisciplinary rather than interdisciplinary, i.e. for insufficient importance to be given to the *integration* of disciplinary perspectives. In this book I am especially interested in the case for 'sociologizing' healthcare ethics. But before saying more on this subject I need to say something about a related issue which has obvious relevance in relation to childhood vaccination. That is, the relevance to healthcare ethics of lay or 'unofficial' knowledge.

In relation to the case under consideration, how should healthcare ethicists respond to those individuals or groups who question the official accounts of the effectiveness or risks of vaccination and present alternative readings of these things? As I indicated in the previous chapter, I would argue that these rival accounts need to be taken very seriously both on their own terms and as a crucially important feature of the context of policy-making. To say that they should be taken seriously on their own terms should not in any way be seen as an endorsement of epistemological relativism. To take them seriously means, in fact, to critically engage with the bases for their truth claims and wherever necessary to find them unsatisfactory, or to dismiss them as plain wrong. However, there should be no presumption that dominant accounts are inherently more valid, and there are good epistemological reasons to listen to the experiences, perceptions and judgements of people who occupy different vantage points. First, 'lived experience' represents in itself a relevant domain of consideration, and second, even from a purely detached or scientific perspective, it is quite possible that communities who are living through certain health experiences will come to conclusions that have the potential to undercut or refine prevailing explanatory frameworks. In short, I would argue that in so far as ethicists have any influence over these things they should help support open discussion and reflection about the relative merits of competing accounts.

When it comes to the policy context of decision-making about vaccination schemes there can simply be no question about the importance of lay perceptions. Clearly the design of such schemes, including the relative importance placed upon elements such as education or public debate depends upon an understanding of lay perceptions; and schemes which are insensitive to the cultural fields in which they are to operate are liable to be hard to defend. Most obviously they risk falling short of the public-health equivalents of 'informed consent', i.e. achievable thresholds for effective communication and public endorsement.

This is one of the reasons that social-science approaches are as necessary to the ethical evaluation of vaccination schemes as the more traditional clinical sciences. What is at stake in vaccination is not merely a bodily intervention but also a social and cultural intervention. To understand such social interventions we have to be ready to draw upon both quantitative and qualitative methods of social inquiry, and we have to live with the kinds of uncertainty and contestability intrinsic to these kinds of inquiry. Furthermore, I want to claim that this need for interdisciplinarity is not just a valuable background resource for healthcare ethics but extends into the core of healthcare ethics. The crucial ethical questions about vaccination schemes, it seems to me, are not of the form 'Is using x or y forms of social influence to underpin such and such a vaccination scheme ethically legitimate in principle?', but of the form 'Is it defensible to implement such and such a vaccination scheme, using x or y forms of social influence under such and such circumstances?' (Later in the chapter I will expand on this point, but I should just stress here that what is in question is not simply whether the relevant set of healthcare goods are realizable under certain circumstances but that the nature and combination of goods realized is a product of circumstances.) Answering this latter kind of context-related practically-oriented question depends upon being able to make complex interpretative readings of specific sets of social expectations, reactions, and relations, of, for example, the varying judgements that citizens make about what is valuable or acceptable from their point of view.[3]

Macro- and micro-contexts. What I am underlining here is the need to ethically appraise vaccination schemes *in context*, by which I mean to include *both* the part they play in the wider health-policy settlement of the state in question *and* the specific ways in which the schemes are embodied in institutions and social relations. The harms and benefits, or rights and wrongs, of a scheme cannot be decided without regard to contextual questions because in a number of respects the contexts constitute the schemes. The defensibility of using school entry as a relatively coercive measure to promote (or 'compel') vaccination depends not only on questions about the real scope for choice-making in such situations, e.g. what other educational arrangements, if any, are open to parents sceptical about vaccination, but also on questions about the overall package of benefits and burdens, or entitlements and obligations, open to the citizens affected. This latter relates to 'the agenda problem' discussed in Chapter 6, i.e. to the question of how far we spread our evaluative gaze. Increasingly policy-makers use the language of 'joined-up thinking' to point to the interrelatedness of various policies and domains of policy. They see, in other words, that it is not sensible to plan or appraise policies in isolation from one another. Healthcare ethicists should aim to be at least as sophisticated as policy-makers in this regard. The defensibility of using social pressure of some kind on parents who are resistant to having

---

[3] The point here is not that what communities find valuable defines what is ethically acceptable; simply that rigorous attempts to make judgements about which policies are ethically acceptable requires attention to the value of policies as they are experienced.

their children vaccinated depends on how it is done—which I will come back to shortly—but it also depends crucially upon how these same parents' preferences and concerns are handled by the same authorities and agencies, or by related agencies, here and in other respects. How much meaningful reciprocity is there between service providers and their clients? This relates both to the 'crude' issue of what citizens get for their 'compliance' with coercive systems, and also to the more subtle issues about the extent to which systems are in the main respectful of, and responsive to, citizens.

These relationships between providers and clients have, of course, to be negotiated and achieved both at the population and the individual level. The nature of the microrelations between 'vaccinators' and 'target families' is, of course, a crucial determinant of the ethical acceptability of schemes. The general argument that it is acceptable, when necessary, to bring some degree of social influence to bear on families, however valid that argument may be, is, in practice, completely insufficient. What is needed is close attention to what in earlier chapters I have called the 'mode' of influence and its practical enactment. That is, for example, how much do individual providers rely upon blanket and heavily paternalistic tactics of 'reassurance and persuasion', or how far do they tailor their relationships in ways that acknowledge the existence of different points of view as well as different needs? As I indicated in the last chapter there are no easy answers to the many ethical dilemmas here, there are some reasons to favour persuasive tactics as well as the more educational and interactive approaches, although as I also pointed out in that chapter, there are arguments in favour of combining persuasive and educational approaches. The acceptability of any potential 'policing tactics' depends upon a realistic assessment of what can be made to happen on the ground, and of course, although this will to a large extent be dependent upon the personal behaviour and style of many separate individuals, the prevailing climates, cultures, and styles of practice are to some extent an appropriate objective of policy-making. (The thought given, and the approach taken, to meeting this objective is itself another factor for ethical appraisal of schemes.)

In this chapter I am principally concerned with methodological rather than substantive questions, but what can I conclude about childhood vaccination schemes and more specifically about the use of strategies of enforcement such as school entry barriers? I would suggest, on the basis of the arguments rehearsed briefly above, that some of these strategies have much to recommend them in principle and should not lightly be ruled out. But I would also want to insist that whether or not they can be defended depends largely upon questions of 'empirical ethics' about whether they can be embodied in sets of practices, and as part of a health-polity settlement, which are both workable and, in turn, ethically defensible. In plain terms this means that the degree of their ethical acceptability will, in practice, vary from case to case, and from polity to polity. This is certainly not a relativistic conclusion; it is simply to acknowledge that what these cases are (the ways that they are socially constituted) varies from instance to instance.

Social and Conceptual Framing

Through the above comments I have tried to illustrate that the three complementary concerns that I have identified for a revised public-health ethics: *broader policy ends and effects, the relevance of different kinds of knowledge, and macro- and micro-contexts* are very closely related. They represent various facets of the way that ethical agendas open out if we move away from an abstract assessment of public-health policies as technical interventions to more grounded analyses of their real embodiment in specific social worlds. This move is made necessary by what I have referred to as the 'social framing' of healthcare and healthcare ethics. Fundamentally it is the necessarily context-specific *embodiment* of health policies that makes narrower conceptions of ethical appraisal inadequate. This is what pushes us away from ethical appraisal as an abstract puzzle about some 'ideal'[4] intervention towards the consideration of the way healthcare goods are practically embodied and enacted. Ethical appraisal involves attention to the full complex of policies and policy effects associated with interventions and this requires a range of empirical sensitivities. Ultimately, however, this shift involves more than the incorporation of various empirical methods into healthcare ethics because it leads us into different forms of reasoning about ethics, including some acceptance of less abstract conceptions of reasonableness. The revised model of public-health ethics that I have sketched places a heavy emphasis on practical judgements, including political judgements, as internal to debates in healthcare ethics. What we are typically faced with is complex judgements about what can be made to work, what can be 'made good', in specific health polities in specific historical, institutional, and cultural moments. In this respect my advocacy of social scientific methods should be seen not as another layer of 'technical knowledge' to feed into the deliberations of ethicists but as an essential part of the practical understanding and deliberation of ethics.[5]

From everything I have said thus far it is hopefully clear why I want to maintain that this 'revised' picture of public-health ethics should be an ingredient of all healthcare ethics. But before continuing I will briefly

---

[4] 'Ideal' here is meant to denote simplified or imagined, rather than 'best possible', although there are often close connections between these readings.

[5] Flyvbjerg (2001) presents a fully worked up defence of this account of social science, i.e. social science as phronesis rather than episteme.

summarize my arguments to this effect. The central point, in a nutshell, is this: policies make practices and, at the same time, practices make policies. In other words, if we want to understand and evaluate the microrelations of healthcare we need to see how they are, in part, produced by the social fields of which they are a part. And, simultanaeously, we need to see how these day-to-day practices serve to make up, sustain, or interrupt, these broader social processes. This is to say no more than I said in the opening chapter, for example, about the ways in which hospital policies on informed consent might help define the possibilities for individual 'consent enactments', and that the lived reality of these multiple 'consent enactments' is what actually determines the de facto hospital policy. But we could interpret this point, which, as I have noted before, is a sociological commonplace that I have used Giddens's 'structuration theory' to indicate, much more widely. Fundamental examples that have run through the book include the ways in which discourses of health promotion, or person-centredness, or evidence-based thinking, and other such reforming discourses, both shape health-professional practice and are mediated by it. The ethical appraisal of such practice, therefore, depends upon an awareness of these two-way processes. It must combine elements of what I have sometimes called internal evaluation and external evaluation. Otherwise such appraisal would quite literally be superficial, looking at the surface interactions and neglecting what lies below the surface and beyond the surface effects. It seems clear to me, for example, that the three 'complementary concerns' that I reviewed above all apply as much to issues in clinical ethics as to the more obviously public-health interventions. To be rigorous in clinical ethics we must see clinical transactions in their social and policy contexts and to be able to study them, and reason about them, in ways that are informed by the social sciences.

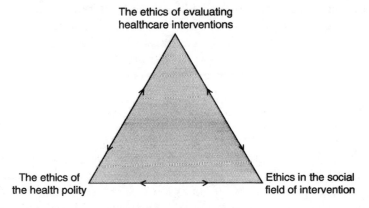

Fig. 3. *The conceptual framing of healthcare ethics.*

Figure 3 is a crude account of what I have called the 'conceptual framing' of issues in healthcare ethics. It is meant to indicate something of the opening out of the ethical agenda that I have been describing. It does not expressly capture the 'social framing' of healthcare, i.e. the respects in which healthcare has to be understood in specific social contexts as an embodied phenomenon which is what entails a role for the social sciences and empirical methods. The figure simply illustrates the interpenetration of three different sets of ethical issues. The corners of the triangle represent different clusters of ethical issues, but there is no suggestion that these issues can be theoretically or practically separated out from one another. Rather the intention is to convey the opposite impression. *The ethics of evaluating healthcare interventions* denotes the fairly circumscribed sets of issues about whether interventions can be justified at all and questions about what can be done to make them as ethically acceptable as possible. In the top corner of the triangle I am imagining that these issues are framed quite narrowly, in the way that I began with the vaccination example above, focusing upon the direct effects of the interventions and the more conspicuous dilemmas they raise. *The ethics of the health polity and broader policy context* denotes questions about the ethical defensibility of the whole health system of which the intervention is a part. These are issues about patterns of policies, for example, about the respective place of markets or state provision, or questions about resource allocation in the system including the emphasis placed upon 'tackling inequalities'. In the bottom-left corner of the triangle I am imagining that these issues are framed quite abstractly, with an emphasis on system- and population-level reasoning and in ways that draw heavily on debates in political philosophy around, for example, theories of deliberative or proced- ural justice. *Ethical issues in the social field of intervention* here denotes the many other questions of ethics that fall outside the scope of healthcare ethics narrowly construed but which are nonetheless implicated in judgements about health policy or specific kinds of healthcare interventions. These questions are too diverse and broad ranging to summarize meaningfully but they would include the kinds of examples I have used before about, for example, sexuality, the family, animal welfare, forms of discrimination or recognition, environmental concerns, etc. They are relevant because health policies and healthcare do not exist in a distinct sphere but cut across social spaces in multiple ways. In some instances, abortion and euthanasia are paradigm examples, the interface between the realm of healthcare and these wider socio-ethical questions is strikingly clear. In many other instances the connections often fall into the background. The ways in which 'institutional discrimination' (on the basis of ethnicity or gender) can be embedded in health policies and forms of organization is perhaps an example of a less overt connection. In the bottom-right of the triangle I imagine these issues are debated in ways that do not highlight the relevance of health policies or healthcare professionals. This is to some extent possible even if we look at paradigm examples. It is possible, for example, to produce an ethical analysis of abortion which leaves on one side questions about the health professionals who might undertake abortions or the institutional contexts of abortion.

What I want to do with this figure is to: (a) point to the whole area of the triangle as the broad way of framing the substantive content of healthcare ethics; (b) use the arrows in the diagram to indicate the interdependency of the three sets of issues and the ways that they merge into one another; and (c) use this simple taxonomy of ethical issues to further illustrate my argument that these dimensions, and the interdependencies between them, apply to the whole field of healthcare ethics and not just to issues in public-health ethics.

Both in relation to conceptual framing and social framing the foci and style of healthcare ethics must 'open out'. Conceptual and social framing apply, as it were, 'at once' and we need to be sensitive to both of them. We can picture Fig. 3 as the top of a triangular column, the depth of which (hidden from view when we consider conceptual-framing alone) represents the social contexts in which the ethical issues arise. This includes a host of factors which shape the way ethical issues are experienced and considered, and the possibilities of their practical resolution including economic and structural constraints, institutional habits and norms, the cultures and subcultures of relevant agents, and so on.

Before concluding this section I want to stress once more that these thoughts about the foci of analyses have substantive as well as methodological implications. The incorporation of a 'public-health' dimension into our thinking about clinical ethics, or to use arguably less contentious terms the incorporation of 'the big picture' into our thinking about locally experienced interpersonal ethics, carries with it a normative load. To think about the big picture is to pay some attention to such things as population health or, more generally, health as a social good. It also serves, as I have claimed in earlier chapters, to sensitize us to questions about the distribution of health goods and 'health opportunities'. This gives rise to a fundamentally important, and deeply complex, substantive ethical question about the ways in which our interpersonal health interactions should be modified to take into account the wider effects of the institutional systems of which they are a part. Specifically, if in some respects they serve to reproduce inequalities in health opportunities then ought we to do what we can to interrupt these processes of reproduction? (This question is just one facet of those more overarching questions about how far those of us who are relatively affluent and powerful should modify our lifestyles so as to further the interests of those who are disadvantaged in various respects.) I will come back to this issue later.

Healthcare Ethics and Social Reflexivity

In the opening chapter I argued that healthcare ethics needs to combine the deliberative elements it draws from applied philosophy with critical elements drawn from a more sociological orientation. This means thinking both about 'how things ought to be' and, at the same time, about 'the social realization of goods and values'. The latter includes what I have called the social and institutional embodiment and concrete enactment of the former. As I have just reiterated, to talk in general terms about desirable ends or underlying principles is worthwhile, but it does not get us very far unless it is allied to a concern with how these things are or might be realized in real social contexts.

It is necessary to spell out what I mean by these remarks a little further because the point I am making is easily misunderstood, or is easily collapsed into two rather different, and less far-reaching, points. I am not simply saying that we need to be concerned with both 'facts' and 'values', that ethicists need to have an accurate 'picture' of the social world on which to base their arguments and recommendations. Nor am I simply making a distinction between 'ethical ends' and 'practical means', where the latter refers to designing policies, strategies, or tactics to get us from A (where we are) to B (where we ought to be). Both these things are essential for healthcare ethics if it is to be an applied ethics as well as a philosophical debate, i.e. it is necessary that ethicists pay some regard to how far their arguments have relevance and to how their conclusions might be practically implemented. However, I am arguing that, in addition to these things, ethicists' arguments and recommendations must be based upon *both* abstract argument *and* a grounded account of healthcare goods and values, because only this synthesis provides a definitive account of what these goods and values can mean, and of how they can be combined. To talk, for example about 'equal access to health care' or about 'respect for autonomy' is to talk about things which have to be understood and managed, in part, in concrete terms. And, finally, I am stressing this not just because goods of this kind have to be socially embodied but also because the 'organizations', e.g. policies, institutional frameworks and social practices, that we design to embody them will inevitably also produce other, frequently unintended and often less visible, 'value effects'. We must, as I have tried to show, ethically appraise not only what is intended by our policies, institutions, and actions but also what is produced by them irrespective of our intentions.

Hence I have taken as my central preoccupation not health-related action per se but the 'value fields' in which actions are set and that shape and influence action. Health policies, healthcare institutions, and the cultures and practices that constitute specific settings embody sets of values: ideals, principles, rules, assumptions, expectations, priorities, etc. of various kinds. Sociologists and social psychologists look to 'norms' of these kinds to help describe and explain patterns of activity, and to illuminate the forms of power or influence and the motivational structures that lie behind them. As I have just said, an understanding of these sorts of social processes is also important to applied ethics, if it is to be 'realistic'. But this has not been the principal focus of this book. I have instead concentrated upon the way that the value field: (a) serves certain 'health agendas' and 'ethical agendas', i.e. embodies conceptions of health-related goods and priorities; (b) reflects a division of ethical labour and assumptions about the distribution of health related responsibilities; and (c) constructs particular healthcare roles which represent distinctive sets of ideals and obligations. More specifically I have been considering the ways in which the value field of health has social agendas of various kinds built into it, and moreover has itself increasingly become the object of attention, through, for example, reforming discourses or managerialism, rather than simply a background phenomenon.

But I am conscious that in arguing for a shift in emphasis from a focus on action to a focus on the social field of action, I could be seen as leaving behind the central point of ethics, and I must resist this interpretation. Whereas sociology, and other social sciences, place great emphasis on the factors that mould or constrain agency, applied ethics rightly places emphasis on the possibilities of agency, on what things ought to be like, or what we ought to do. These ethical questions only make sense if they are based on assumptions about us approaching the social world as agents with responsibility for shaping it, and certainly not merely as products of 'social forces'. So I am not arguing for a total shift in focus away from action but only for a shift in emphasis. The idea is not that action is neglected but that it is properly set in its social context. Indeed, this is exactly what is aspired to in most social science, much of which is opposed to crude models of social determinism. As I discussed in relation to structuration theory, the object, more often than not, is to account for both 'social forces' and 'agency' and for the relationships between them.

This dual focus is, I am suggesting, as important to applied ethics as it is to sociology. Those with an interest in applied ethics have to avoid two kinds of foolishness about the nature of the social world. On the one hand there is the foolishness of supposing that the social world can be magically 'condensed' from their airy conclusions about how things ought to be. On the other hand there is the foolishness of supposing that the social and institutional frameworks that make up the arena of action provide a fixed backdrop to ethical analysis rather than part of its subject matter. What is needed is an outlook that sees social and institutional frameworks as relatively stable 'conveyors' of social values and 'shapers' of action, and at the same time as reproduced by, and amenable to revision by, social actors and their value choices. It is precisely this dual focus which I have tried to capture at various points by arguing for a combination of internal and external evaluation, i.e. a combination of those evaluative stances which operate inside specific social frameworks and stances that attempt to stand back from these frameworks.

I do not want to suggest that the call for this dual focus is especially novel nor that it involves something esoteric or technical. Indeed, it merely reflects my opening discussion about the increasingly widespread existence of forms of social reflexivity. After all, social reflexivity is really nothing more than the ability both to occupy one's situation and also to be able to see it as contingent and open to change. Also, in my discussion of 'the agenda problem' in Chapter 6, I made it clear that this dual focus is sometimes explicitly addressed in healthcare ethics. It would, in fact, be difficult to conceive of an approach to healthcare ethics which did not somehow wrestle with this problem, because we are continuously forced to think about which 'parameters' to adopt and which to question. All I am arguing is that sociological perspectives on the construction and relative determinacy of the social world should form a greater part of the toolkit, and the self-consciousness, of applied ethicists. I certainly do not want to play down the centrality of action or ethical responsibility, I intend the opposite. I simply wish to ensure that healthcare ethics does not rely on socially disembedded, and therefore misleading, conceptions of action or responsibility.

In the following chapter I will illustrate my responses to the agenda problem in a little more depth. To conclude this chapter I will offer a somewhat sweeping summary of my stance. Hopefully the illustrations and reflections that follow will help make it seem a plausible one. Generally speaking, I would argue, we each have some responsibility to divide our attention between our immediate 'role-related' obligations and the wider evaluation and construction of the social frameworks that define these roles and associated 'ethical positions'. One aspect of this broader responsibility, and an aspect that I have given considerable prominence to, is seeking to understand the value field of health-related action: of the ways in which health-related goods are socially constructed and produced, and of the scope for changing these things. There is undoubtedly a great deal of indeterminacy about what degrees or kinds of social change are possible but, I would suggest, this indeterminacy demands an ethical and not merely an epistemological response. That is, I contend, we all have a duty to challenge assumptions about who is responsible for whose health, and about what can and cannot be done to make a difference to people's health experiences.

12

Making the Health Agenda

To conclude the book I want to look at the shape of the health agenda. In other words I want to consider some of the health-policy choices we face, whether as legislators, managers, health professionals, or as individual citizens. As in earlier chapters I am not especially interested in trying to decide the substantive questions of health policy and healthcare ethics, i.e. I am not trying to determine the choices we should make. Rather I am interested in asking about what some of the choices are. Where and what is the scope for action? And what sorts of things are at stake? Of course, it is important to be wary when talking loosely about a collective 'we' who are facing issues in health policy or healthcare ethics. It is not merely that different individuals and groups have different interests and perspectives, but also that they are differently positioned as regards to both the power and knowledge required to address issues. However, as I have argued above and wish to underscore again, we should be equally wary of assuming any firm separation between 'decision-makers' and others. At each level, whether specific professional–client encounters, the construction of institutional policies, or the shaping or enactment of public-health policy, there are opportunities for participation. I have already argued for the central importance of a revivified health education to underpin greater participation in decision-making processes; whilst at the same time I accept, for the reasons rehearsed in Chapter 3, that participation will often be in the agenda-setting or deliberative phases of decision-making rather than in the executive ones.

In talking about the choices we face I mean mainly to refer to choices about healthcare 'philosophies' rather than choices about healthcare technologies, although I will say a little about the latter in passing. Much has been written about cutting-edge developments and innovations in clinical research and science and, what is more, these topics do provide a valuable medium through which to explore important philosophical questions about healthcare. But I have nothing significant to add to that literature here. Instead, as I explained in the opening chapter, I am essentially interested in issues and challenges that have been opened up by other sets of developments associated with 'late modernity', developments I have summarized as the 'social turn' in the construction of the health agenda.

In the last chapter I wrote about the social field of healthcare both as something which is 'given' and as something which we can critique and influence. This relates to the two contrasting senses in which the health agenda is 'set', i.e. is 'fixed' or is 'made'. I now want to explore the relationship between these two senses by looking at a couple of examples. Throughout the book I have referred to two major, interacting, sets of public-health policy drivers: biomedicine and economics. These provide the basis for the next two sections. Crudely speaking the norms of biomedicine powerfully shape the 'content' of healthcare, its purposes and internal practices. The complex of economic norms and pressures, which are manifest in debates about budgets and priorities, and about markets of various kinds, help to shape the forms of healthcare organization. But these two sets of factors interact or, to put it another way, the distinction between 'content' and 'form', or between 'practice' and 'organization' cannot really be sustained. Biomedicine encompasses structures as well as cultures, and as well as embodying the discourses of medical science, including the contesting and reforming discourses I have focused upon, it links into the economic power of the medical profession and the wider health economy. Similarly forms of economic organization and the competitive/comparative pressures on healthcare providers do not simply provide parameters for provision but, as has been explored in various places above, penetrate into the forms and possibilities of care.

The Drive of Globalization

It is only sensible for us to think about our hopes, fears, and plans in the context of the political and economic infrastructures that underpin our lives and the socio-cultural movements which shape our understandings, experiences, and choices. Also from the point of view of any individual, especially the very many who have little power, it is only natural to think of these contextual factors as overwhelming forces to which they are subject in just the same way that they are subject to plate tectonics or earthquakes. However, it is also important to see that there is, as I have been stressing, some 'degree of play' in the social world, i.e. that social structures and movements do not completely determine actions, nor even entirely determine the 'option sets' of individuals and, once again, are themselves susceptible to human intentions. To illustrate this I am starting with an unquestionably large-scale example, debates about the nature and direction of 'globalization'.

Globalization is obviously a big subject, and one which cannot be treated adequately here. It is a name used for a whole range of phenomena, and the existence and significance of some of these phenomena are hotly contested.

The central axis of the globalization thesis is an economic one but this is closely linked to contentions about broader political and socio-cultural change. The economic thesis points to the existence of a new regime of free-trade competition on a worldwide scale. A global free market, supported by new technologies, and a market which through competition in wages and tax costs leads to increased mobility of capital, goods, services, and labour. Alongside this central thesis are related arguments about the extent to which global markets are deepening or ameliorating patterns of global inequality (Sivanandan, 1989; Massey, 1999). The political implications of these trends are often presented as of great magnitude and importance: (a) there is much talk of the relative decline of the power of nation states and governments as compared to economically powerful regions within states and more powerful supranational organizations; (b) tax competition is seen as producing more pressure to curtail or reduce public spending or, at least, to closely regulate the efficient use and prudent stewardship of public monies. The socio-cultural dimensions of globalization are perhaps the most difficult to specify but include competing theories about: (a) the growth of global products and services and trends of cultural homogenization including the spread of the Anglo-American language; and (b) the increase in hybrid cultural identities through population movements and through new consumer identities which give global trends and products 'local referencing' (Appadurai, 1996).

Theses about globalization provide a paradigm case of the ways in which the social field of action is seemingly generated by forces which completely transcend individual agency. For example, the factors which I have presented as producing the reconstruction of health-professional roles and subjectivities are closely linked to these globalization accounts. Here I am talking about such factors as: the extensive penetration of competitive/ comparative cultures, increasingly in the public as well as in the private sector; the ubiquitous pressures on cost-control and for efficiency-related measures and measurements; and the rise of managerialist structures and climates as a means of controlling professional behaviours and expenditures. On this reading there is, for instance, a direct connection between a health professional's frustration with some new managerial performance indicator and the 'world historical forces' of globalization. More generally, many of the debates associated with the increasing influence of market thinking and practices in healthcare, in regions around the world, overlap with debates about globalization. They provide some of the most fundamental questions and concerns about the nature and direction of healthcare. Should the nations of Western Europe, for example, be worried about the increasing role of private-sector organizations and cultures in the funding or provision of healthcare, and the possible deleterious effects of increased corporate power, competitive pressures, and market-related commodification? Or should they, at least to some degree, be celebrating the relative emancipation of healthcare consumers from the stranglehold of the state and professional paternalism?

But, whatever the balance of our thinking on these matters, what is an individual health professional, or an individual citizen, supposed to do in the wake of such massive global forces? This is meant, for the most part, as a rhetorical question. However, merely to develop my theme, I will begin to construct a response to it.

The crux of what can be said in response to this question is that: (1) it is simply wrong to think of globalization as a 'force', especially when this suggests something uncontrollable and overwhelming; and (2) however overbearing some of these economic changes appear to be there is always scope for agency at various levels from the local level and so to speak 'upwards'. A further look at the globalization literature shows why the 'force' kind of image is misleading. Hall, for example, asks us to be sceptical about the reification of globalization into a 'single uncontradictory phenomenon which gives rise to inevitable outcomes everywhere and is uncontrollable by nation states either individually or as a collective force' (Hall, 1998: 11). What is being encouraged here is not merely a view about an empirical knowledge claim ('Is "globalization" happening or not?') but also an ethical and political attitude ('What ought we to do about changes in world markets?'). Furthermore this critical and ethical stance is lent support by other scholars who question the view of globalization as summarized by Hall, i.e. what has been called 'the strong globalization thesis' (Hirst and Thompson, 1999). There are, in brief, two clusters of reasons to be sceptical about the picture of globalization as overwhelming. First, as Hirst and Thompson set out in depth, there are many reasons to doubt that the changes to international political economy are either as new, as pervasive, or as uncontrollable as the strong thesis suggests. For example, they argue that the G3, the three major economic powers of Europe, Japan, and North America, have the power, especially if they coordinate policy, to exert significant governance pressures over markets, that global markets are simply not beyond regulation and control. In turn this highlights the potential role of political action by powerful government agents and by those that can influence them. Second, even if we were to accept that economic processes can be regulated only within very narrow limits, this does not in any case undercut the place of individual agency because economic processes are themselves mediated by agency. Consumers of goods and services clearly have some degree of choice about what they consume. Market advocates may exaggerate the idea of consumer sovereignty as both the mechanism and the legitimation of markets, but no one could seriously deny any place for choice in economic life. This is why one of the trends sometimes linked to globalization is 'individualization', i.e. an increased opportunity and emphasis on individuals being able to 'pick and mix' the goods and services they value, consume, and through which they construct their own hybrid identities (Appadurai, 1996). More generally, whether working in, or engaging with, either private or public-sector organizations there is always some 'freedom of manoeuvre' about how economic or other considerations are interpreted and dealt with.

To repeat, I am not trying to make a contribution to the scholarly debates about globalization here, I am only using globalization as a paradigm case of a 'powerful social force' and underlining the importance of not being seduced by this kind of imagery. Whatever the merits of the case for a stronger or weaker globalization thesis there are both empirical and ethical reasons to emphasize the opportunity for action that makes a difference to globalization. In addition the global is always mediated through the local, through particular contexts, settings, and agents. This means that although most individual agents cannot expect to make a significant difference to change at a global level there is no reason to rule out individuals' potential role as part of some collective body, and, just as important, there is every reason to highlight their potential influence on their immediate environments. I would argue that this analysis applies to any kind of structural pressure or social movement, however large or small scale.

The Drive of Biomedicine

Although I have highlighted many of the 'diffusing' trends that have moderated the influence of narrower medical models, there is no doubting the influential role of biomedical discourse in the construction of the health agenda. Without repeating the arguments of the previous section, I should start by noting the fallacy of reifying 'the medical model', as if it were an independent and unified social force that has captured the field irrespective of people's preferences. It is important to see that reference to biomedicine picks out: (a) a complex cluster of overlapping, and sometimes competing, social processes and practices; and (b) a set of things which are in many respects straightforwardly valuable and which, very often, immediately reflect people's needs and wants. It is, I suggest, absurd to treat 'medicine' or 'the medical model' as purely pejorative expressions.

Nonetheless, reference to the medical model or to biomedical discourse is often made with critical intent to capture certain 'narrow' tendencies in healthcare. 'Narrow' here implies something like an unmoderated, scientistic instrumentalism, which might, for example, lead to an overemphasis on disease rather than illness, or on cure rather than care. Indeed, this sort of thing provides the central plank of innumerable critical readings of healthcare. In the light of this well-known story how can we best understand the continuing power of biomedical perspectives and how can we best engage with them? I am asserting that here, as with the case of globalization, we need to bring together sociological and ethical perspectives. We need, that is, to combine a sociological interest in explanation and critique with a philosophical interest in ethical appraisal and deliberation. Although I will not attempt to offer to review them here there is much to be gained from historical or sociological accounts of the power of medicine. Such accounts offer invaluable material to make use of and synthesize. I have already pointed to the undeniable practical efficacy of much medicine, to the fact that it connects with real needs and demands. But this factor intersects with many others: there is the prestige and status of the medical sciences; there is the power inherent in the relationship between the clinical expert and the vulnerable patient; there are the ideologies of professionalism and the collective social power of such a major professional group; and there are the commercial interests which sustain healthcare systems and resource use, etc. The interaction between these and other factors and the general feature of 'social inertia' which makes social structures, cultures, traditions, and practices 'sticky', i.e. makes them adhere in places which may not be ideal, make it unsurprising that medical power is the subject of so much criticism. The value field of healthcare is sometimes shaped by norms and interests which can be judged, with good reason, to be short-sighted, wrong-headed, or unresponsive. And this helps to account for instances where we might find, for example, excessive paternalism or self-interestedly motivated 'overtreatment'.

An understanding of the power of biomedical discourse is useful, for example, when we come to consider the appraisal of new medical technologies. New technologies in screening, diagnosis, and treatment, whether advances in traditional approaches or the introduction of novel approaches in fields such as biotechnology, are the subject of constant and high-profile controversy. On both sides of these controversies there are countless examples of 'knee-jerk' thinking. On the one hand there is the extraordinary persistence of a Luddite mentality, a mind-set that resists the disruption of the taken for granted, the familiar, or the 'natural', and which is fuelled by fears of science-fiction horror stories. On the other hand there is what is sometimes labelled 'the technological imperative', a presumption that progress necessarily flows from technical advance, and that the fact that something may be technically possible itself provides a prima facie reason to do it. I would argue that both these sets of prejudices arise from the influence of prominent currents in biomedical discourse. To the extent that the medical model can be informed by a narrow scientistic instrumentalism, more or less married to commercial interests, it is likely to support a presumption such as the technological imperative. And to the extent that this scientistic instrumentalism is experienced as alien and unresponsive to existing life-worlds then this is bound to provoke a defensive backlash that can take Luddite forms.

Health-technology assessment, I suggest, needs to start from a recognition of these countervailing sets of prejudices and the ways they arise. This means that particular technologies should not only be appraised on their own terms, 'Does it do what it claims to do and is this a good thing?', but in the context of the wider sets of goods and values that they reinforce or neglect. On occasions this sort of evaluation may well provide strong reasons for being sceptical about new technologies; reasons with much more warrant than a knee-jerk dismissal. For example the steady extension of the use of drug therapies in the name of the emotional well-being of children and adolescents may well be a case where the biomedical drive ought to be resisted.

But uncovering and critiquing the value field of healthcare is not enough. We need to use such explanations and critical readings as a starting point for asking how things might be different in both principle and practice. As I have said biomedical discourse serves an important set of purposes and is organized around an important set of goods. And whilst we must look to how some of its deficiencies or unwanted side-effects might be repaired at both macro- and micro-levels, we have to do so without supposing that we can step outside of social reality. We have to find not only the right set of principles and ideals but also a suitable set of social mechanisms to realize them. The ultimate object of our deliberations must be the social and institutional embodiment of our ethical ideals and principles. This is why I have been arguing we need to combine a 'sociological ethics' with a philosophical ethics. To stress what I have called the social construction of health goods is not in any way to play down the importance of purely theoretical or even speculative versions of applied healthcare ethics. Rather what I am suggesting is that deliberative ethics, however speculative it is, will often be improved if it arises from a careful consideration of the social field of healthcare and health policy. And that, in addition to argumentative rigour, one of the dimensions of rigour that has relevance for deliberative ethics is how well its premises and conclusions are connected with the social contexts to which it claims relevance.

Persons and Patterns: Competing Ideals in Healthcare

Making the purposes and principles, and associated interests and motivations, that are socially embedded in healthcare more explicit is a necessary foundation for broader and better public education and debate. But in addition we need an open-ended and wide-ranging debate about healthcare ideals. Policy-makers, health professionals, and citizens all have a role to play in developing critically informed perspectives on healthcare purposes and ideals both: (a) to inform macro-level policy reform and (b) to use as yardsticks against which to assess specific healthcare practices.

The reforming discourses and other trends that I have lumped together in discussion of the diffusion of the health agenda indicate some of the elements that a reimagined healthcare system might have to combine. There are so many competing considerations here that it would be foolish even to attempt to map them all. I have concentrated on a few key dimensions of contest-ation, and especially on some of the balances between individual-oriented and population-oriented conceptions of healthcare. Other dimensions in-clude: the balance between professionally initiated, future-oriented preven-tion or health promotion and more responsive treatment of expressed needs; the balance between treatment interventions or 'cure' and person-regarding 'care'; and the related balance, whether at the individual or population level, between a biomedically defined clinical agenda and a broader interpretation of 'health' or well-being.

In order to illustrate some of these fundamental tensions underlying health policy I will return to just two elements: the idea of person-centred care and the inequalities reflected in disease and death rates. I have chosen these two elements not only for illustrative reasons but also because I believe that they are absolutely crucial axes in future health-policy debates. They both repre-sent departures from a certain traditional and narrow conception of the medical model, and for that reason I have previously discussed them both as features of a more diffused health agenda; but they are departures which seem, at least in some respects, to go in contrasting directions.

I have already written, in Part I of the book, about the different facets of person-centred care, the interests in holism, specificity, and agency. Here I want to say a little more about another facet that is closely related to each of these, namely an interest in the meaning of health and illness experiences. I have deliberately argued for, and used, a conception of health that is, in part, understood in relation to illness, to the *experiences* of disease or disability, i.e. to the significance these things have in relation to an individ-ual's biography, self-identity, and social identity. Placing 'meanings' at the centre of healthcare is undoubtedly an essential component of person-cent-redness, otherwise we seem to be dealing with bodies rather than full persons who are, roughly speaking, constituted by meanings as well as by matter. Many of the health-related goods that I have discussed arise from this fact. I have talked, for example, about the value of knowledge, of understanding, and of support in making sense of one's experiences. I have also talked about the goods related to respect or recognition. In most instances respect cannot simply be a generalized regard for another person's value or dignity but entails some recognition of, and attention to, the 'point of view' of the individual concerned. In the normal case, that is, recognition includes recognition of the subjective standpoint, including both individual perspectives and the cultural worlds that partly constitute subjectivity.

All of this is embraced in most recent models of healthcare. Within both medicine and nursing there are many authors playing up the importance of practitioners relating to, and responding to, the life-worlds of patients and others. This general concern has, for example, spawned two broad and cross-cutting sets of professional interests, an interest in lay cultures and an interest in personal narratives. Here both culture and narrative can be interpreted narrowly or broadly, as relating to the specific cultural resources or stories that are used to make sense of immediate illness experiences, or as relating to the very broad cultural or biographical frameworks against which health and illness experiences are understood and managed. It should be obvious why these concerns represent a major component in the diffusion of the health agenda. They raise very large challenges for health professionals and, therefore, make similarly large demands on healthcare resources. It is not merely that health professionals may need to be sensitive to, and ready to differentiate between, different cultural readings of disease or disability, e.g. readings influenced by religion or ethnicity, but also that they may need to be responsive to the absolutely specific interpretations and concerns of individuals. This latter has the potential to be a limitless task, as there is no clear limit to individuals' need for recognition and dialogue as they come to terms with their unfolding experiences. Given that the reflexive construction of one's own identity and subjectivity is widely seen as a characteristic good of late modernity (Giddens, 1991; Taylor, 1992), it is unsurprising to see the acknowledgment of this good practice, and associated ones, gaining ground in health-policy discourses.

The growing prominence of policy debates about inequalities in patterns of morbidity and mortality, discussed in Chapter 5, is in some respects[1] a contrasting component of the diffused health agenda. This is obviously a population-oriented interest and in particular an interest in whether the distribution of people's life opportunities, in relation to certain basic goods, is fair. Expressed in these terms, however, it is an interest which is effectively blind to the person-specific elements of ill-health and to the realm of subjectivity. These two components of diffusion both present us with fundamental ethical demands; and the tensions between them reflect what are arguably the central tensions in ethical thinking. We are obliged to treat

---

[1] The importance of inequalities in recognition, discussed in Ch. 5, indicates that these two sets of concerns can overlap.

individuals with respect and, to some extent, this means dealing with people 'on their own terms'. But we are also obliged to treat people fairly, and not to allow our involvement with some individuals to undercut our response to the ethical claims of others.

The conflict I have constructed between attention to life-worlds and attention to health opportunities is not meant to suggest some easy resolution, even at the level of principle. I do not want to present an interest in life-worlds as simply a kind of luxury to be contrasted, for example, with the premature deaths of the disadvantaged. Speaking for myself for a moment, I do not want to die earlier than I need to, but I would definitely hesitate to postpone death if I knew that it would be at the cost of dying uncared for and alone. As I have noted before, death is not always trumps in value disputes. For most people the opportunity to continue living is valuable to the extent that life is experienced as valuable and meaningful, and health professionals and other health-carers certainly have some part to play in helping people make sense of their experience and maintain a hold on the value of life.

As policy-makers, health professionals, or citizens how far should we be arguing for health policies and practices to be based around individual life-worlds or around fairer health opportunities? In this section heading I have labelled these two concerns as 'competing ideals', but there is actually no reason to suppose that they are incompatible at the level of principle. Any health polity is likely to attach some importance to both of these things. The tensions between these contrasting goods and other health-related goods arise because policies and practices will inevitably be more effective in some directions than in others. So how ought we to address this question about competing ideals in the design of healthcare? For the moment I am simply floating this question and leaving aside complications about the extent to which the levers which affect these things are under our control. Ignoring these crucial complications, what do we think healthcare ought to be for?

This can be seen as an example—albeit a rather broadly conceived and abstract example—of the priority-setting problem. Instead of asking which kinds of healthcare interventions ought to be made available within certain resource constraints or, slightly more generally, asking about how to divide our resources between different kinds of interventions such as treatment or prevention, we are asking about how to determine the relative weight we attach to the different possible ends of healthcare or health policy. Indeed the language of, and debates about, priority-setting should perhaps be understood as one of the main ways in which philosophical disagreements about healthcare come to the surface of policy analysis. The surface importance of priority-setting discussions gives debate about the proper direction of healthcare the prominence it merits, but it also tends to obscure much of what is at stake behind reductionist and technicist rhetoric about such notions as 'maximizing outcomes'. Ultimately priority-setting is not about weighing and comparing medical interventions but about asking if we cannot get everything from healthcare, what do we want to get from it?

Arguably Dan Callahan has done more than anyone else to press home this underlying question. He contrasts what he calls the 'infinity model' of healthcare with a finite model.[2] The former seeks 'unending biological knowledge and technological innovation' with the aim of eradicating disease and eliminating suffering. The latter by contrast: accepts mortality and human finitude (e.g. something like present developed-country lifespans are acceptable), tolerates limits to, and rationing of, healthcare, and prizes care almost as highly as cure and public health at least as much as individual health. This finite model, as constructed here by Callahan, is, he argues, 'seemingly on the decline in the United States and some Western European countries but still visible in central Europe and much of the developing world' (2003: 8). This distinction between the infinity and the finite models is a simple one, but for that very reason is a powerful resource for thinking about, and evaluating, health-policy directions. Callahan uses it to force those of us in the most affluent health polities to question the real cost of the drive for what he calls 'open-ended medical progress'. This, as I have said, represents the real priority-setting agenda.

However, I would want to add some extra dimensions to this contrast between the finite and the open-ended. It seems to me, in fact I have been trying to illustrate throughout the book, that open-endedness is multifaceted. It is not simply that the quest for technological innovation, for new and more medicines and treatments, is open-ended. The same applies to the possibilities of 'caring', the demands of personal and cultural recognition, and to the various imperatives of public health. The diffusion of the health agenda opens up each of these things in ways that are potentially limitless. As I indicated above there is no clear limit to the level of 'individual recognition' that can be offered as individuals negotiate every moment and contour of their shifting health experiences. In certain areas of palliative care, for example, very close attention is given to the detailed texture of day-to-day experience and sense-making. In principle there is no reason such attention could not be afforded in many other instances and areas. Equally health professionals and healthcare institutions could indefinitely extend their responsiveness to the perspectives of diverse cultural groups and the ways in which cultural memberships inform and constitute the experience, meaning, and significance of health and healthcare. Similarly, the demands of (often conflicting) public-

---

[2] This is a thesis developed in a number of publications but the quotes that follow are taken from the 'Medicine and the Market' book proposal (2003). I am very grateful to Dan Callahan for sight of, and discussions about, this proposal and some draft chapters.

health agendas are apparently boundless, whether this refers to the redistributive and recognitional dimensions of inequality, discussed in Chapter 5, or the open-ended demands for ever more health promotion reviewed in Chapter 4. In short, the tensions between the infinite and the finite are not really those between the technological imperative on the one hand and a concern with care or public health on the other; practical lines of finitude have to be drawn both across and within each of these concerns.

Philosophical analyses of priority-setting recognize these fundamental tensions in debating the competing evaluative frameworks for determining priorities. Indeed, the fact that not only the value of substantive priorities but also the frameworks of prioritization are inherently contested has led many philosophers to switch emphasis from thinking about 'principles of allocation' to thinking about 'principles of deliberation' (Daniels and Sabin, 1998; Holm, 1998). The rationale for this switch of emphasis being that because there is no decisive (and certainly no neutral) means of determining the former in the abstract then we need to find practical and fair procedures for settling priorities through collective deliberation.[3]

As I argued in Chapter 10 I see no areas of debate or deliberation from which anyone should be excluded. Although not everyone will be interested in debates about competing frameworks of evaluation, there is no reason to confine 'members of the public' to the role of being consulted, or to playing a part in some specific deliberative process. There is no need for rigid boundaries between 'experts' and others here. What, however, is needed when these debates have practical outcomes, are social mechanisms through which what are deemed to be acceptable standards of reasoning or deliberation are underpinned. As I argued in Chapter 3 this does entail the construction of appropriate forms of social authority, but these can be constructed so as to allow for relatively more rather than less inclusion in decision-making.

Realizing Health as a Social Good

In this final section of the book I want to pull together some of the threads by reflecting on the question of health purposes and priorities a little further. The foci of the previous section, 'life worlds' and 'fair opportunities', were chosen to exemplify the tension, which has run through this book, between more person-oriented and more population-oriented perspectives. In this section I want to acknowledge the difficulty of orienting healthcare to either *persons* or *patterns*.

---

[3] Following on from the discussion about social reflexivity, I would want to note the importance of these debates about principle being conducted in conjunction with an analysis of the way principles are mediated by macro- and micro-political discourses (Wirtz *et al.*, 2003).

As I explained in Chapter 7 there are a number of different ways of reading the distinction between 'persons' and 'populations' because there are different facets and interpretations of the two concepts. We can emphasize more person-specific or more generic kinds of goods; we can emphasize forms of partiality or impartiality, we can emphasize the needs of an individual or the needs of a population: these distinctions are related in various ways but they are different distinctions. Engagement with life-worlds is a facet of person-centredness, as I have said, because it is about the full recognition of persons, but there is no reason to equate a population perspective with a completely 'impersonal' standpoint, where 'impersonal' implies a neglect of subjectivity. Population-oriented values in healthcare, assuming they are ethically defensible, will reflect some model of impartiality, but they can also reflect a concern with culture and subjectivity. It is simply that the more we move to a population-orientation the less fine-grained and open-ended the engagement with *specific* persons can be; and the more likely we are to adopt what I am calling an impersonal standpoint. But an orientation towards *both* the elements I picked out above, towards both persons and patterns, is part of what I referred to in Chapter 1 as 'the social turn' in healthcare. These orientations represent the widening and deepening features of the diffused health agenda, a concern with the psychosocial realm and the interpersonal and a concern with the determinants and patterns of disease.

In other words the interest in life-worlds and fair opportunities both illustrate the ways in which healthcare increasingly deals with the individual body as part of the 'social body'. In this final section of the book I will rely on this somewhat simplistic distinction between a kind of 'clinical individualism' on the one hand and more socially aware approaches to health on the other. I should start by stressing that this is essentially an ideal typical distinction being employed for heuristic reasons. What I have to say here about 'individualism' thus refers to the potential neglect of the widening and deepening tendencies, to giving an undue emphasis to individual bodies in ways that fail to reflect both whole persons and wider patterns. I readily concede that what I want to say here, because it relies on an exaggerated distinction, is liable to fall into the trap of criticizing a 'straw-man' position. But I still believe that there is some value in trading in these general ideal types, and I say this partly because I believe they reflect important features that have a real presence and considerable influence in health-policy discourses.

Both the market form and the clinical tradition of medicine have a tendency to treat health as a good which is defined, 'produced', and 'enjoyed' at the individual level. And to the extent that these discourses are dominant in healthcare, and are combined in ways that arguably reinforces their individualizing tendencies, then individualism plays a major role in the value field of health policy. What is more, I would argue, there are influential approaches to health policy that further embed these tendencies in the social construction of health. These approaches are captured in the idea of a 'policy science' (Fay, 1975), an approach to policy-making and evaluation that looks to identify those policies which are most effective in delivering specified ends. In much policy construction and debate this largely 'technicist' model is assumed. According to the most naïve policy-science approaches the job of policy is simply to identify the best means of achieving our valued ends, where the ends are derived from our choices and/or our 'social and political philosophy'. In this case this would mean finding the most effective means of delivering health outcomes to individuals according to some specified set of allocative criteria. Within this kind of framework both clinical biomedicine and the market can be seen essentially as tools, as relatively neutral means for achieving the ends of health policy.

It should be clear why I think this is a seriously misleading and, in many respects, damaging picture. First, I would maintain that there are no clear boundaries between health goals and other goals, or between a health sector and other sectors. Second, as I have tried to underline, the policies and practices that promote or underpin health are not neutral but themselves embody various kinds of health-related goods and other social goods. I will briefly review each of these points.

The 'boundary' issue is of absolutely fundamental importance to analysing health and health policy. To put it plainly: healthcare serves other ends than those of health, and other social processes and policies bring about a wide range of health-related goods, including central biomedical ends such as the prevention of disease and death. And specifying the goals of healthcare is impossible without addressing the question of what the specific contribution of healthcare is to well-being. Brülde (2001), for example, has identified a goal-set for medicine which includes a range of different goals that are causally and conceptually interrelated and which, he argues, cannot be reduced to some simpler set. He identifies the following goals as making up the goal set of medicine: promoting function, curing or preventing disease, promoting quality of life, saving and prolonging life, supporting coping, creating 'less handicapping' environments, and supporting child development. Although what he calls the 'final goals' of medicine are summarized in two of these, i.e. *promoting quality of life* and *saving and prolonging life*, these two goals can only be understood as the goals of medicine, he argues, by considering their links to the other goals through which medicine meets them. Considered out of this context the two final goals could belong to many activities, including eating and exercising or military defence.

There are equally important difficulties in distinguishing between 'the goals' of healthcare or well-being and the activities and practices designed to support them, i.e. there are conceptual problems inherent in trying to separate the purposes of these fields of activity from the activities themselves. In other words the goods that healthcare practices serve are partly internal to the practices. (A nurse comforting a distressed patient is not generically 'promoting quality of life' but is comforting a distressed patient.)

To summarize: it is very difficult to disentangle the goals of health and well-being, and it is very difficult to disentangle goals and practices. This means that the problem for the would-be policy-maker interested in under-pinning health-related goods is not simply one of prioritizing health amongst a basket of goods. It is not simply about the question, *'How can health be weighed against other goods?'* (Other aspects of well-being, or other values which might be undermined in the pursuit of health.) But it is also about at least two other questions: *'How far should health outcomes be pursued through healthcare systems and institutions or through other broader policies?'* and *'What are the other goods (beyond narrow health outcomes) internal to healthcare or health-policy activities and how important are these in their own right?'* These extra dimensions complicate social and political decision-making about health considerably. Instead of thinking purely about some 'separate' health sector, how it should be funded, managed, and regulated, what its guiding ideals and principles should be, etc., social and political agents with an interest in health have to consider the whole of society. This precludes, for example, making easy distinctions between the organizing principles and values pertaining to health-related action and those that apply elsewhere. It may be, for example, that the welfare-state model of a 'market insulated' healthcare sector in a broadly market-based society can be defended. But it certainly cannot be defended on the straightforward basis that 'health is a separate matter'.

To reiterate, I am suggesting that a combination of factors contribute to a strongly influential mind-set in which health is treated as if it was a kind of separate medical commodity to be delivered to individuals. Having noted that this picture entails too strong a distinction between healthcare and other things, I will briefly add some comments about my second concern, namely that individualistic discourses can seriously obscure the ways in which health can usefully be seen as a social good. I distinguished a number of these in Chapter 2. There are, I think, three main dimensions here, which can be variously combined: (1) it makes sense to talk about the 'collective health' of a group or population. At its simplest and least contentious this means an 'overview' of the health of the individuals concerned using aggregate and distributive measures of disease; (2) some healthcare or health-related goods (and these goods would also be reflected in broader conceptions of health itself) are social in nature, i.e. they involve forms of mutuality or solidarity. Indeed, on some conceptions of health, even comparatively narrow ones, it is not really tenable to split off either the meaning or importance of 'health experiences' from the interpersonal arenas in which they take place; and (3) both health and the distribution of health have 'social determinants'. Overall, what these elements point to is the overwhelmingly large number of ways in which different people's lives, health status, and health experiences are interrelated. These myriad relations and mutual implications operate both at the level of causality and at the level of the meaning of our experience.

The fact that it is possible, and that it can be useful, to talk about health as a social good does not, of course, mean that it is always wise to talk in these terms. There are many real disputes to be had about the extent to which these three dimensions of 'socialness' could, without significant loss, be translated into individualist terms. Furthermore, there is the question of the extent to which, even if they do capture something important that evades a more individualist language, they can and ought to displace an individualist model of health provision. I am not going to say more about these disputes. I have already indicated often enough that I think some degree of shift in dominant discourses to a less individualist construction of health is happening and that it is broadly to be welcomed. I have also indicated that evaluating these shifts is far from straightforward and that there are costs to consider as well as benefits.

What I do want to say is that the recognition of the depth and density of our interrelatedness ought to prompt widespread reflection about the correct division of ethical labour in matters of health. We now understand enough about the way in which health is socially realized for us to be asking searching questions about the respective roles and responsibilities of health professionals, 'official policy-makers', and other citizens. As I have argued these questions must encompass a concern with the ways that structures and cultures shape the value field of healthcare and the ways in which we can, individually and collectively, actively construct the value field. This will help us to understand why certain things are debated and even accomplished whilst other things fall off the agenda. For example, as things stand it is, I would suggest, much easier to give person-centred care a prominent place on the health agenda (whatever the complexion of the health polity) than it is to give prominence to inequalities in death and disease. This is not, I think, because those with an interest in health believe that inequalities are less important, but largely because addressing inequalities takes us beyond the relatively safe frame of healthcare.

Recognizing the social construction of both health and ethical agendas should also teach us that public-policy debates about health cannot simply 'follow on from' independent debates about social and political philosophy. Practical policy analysis and social philosophy are interdependent activities. This is because health and other related goods can only be understood and valued in the context of the social fields and social relationships that embody them. For this reason I would suggest that health-policy analysis has substantial importance for political philosophy. There is no point talking grandly about commitments to equal respect or equal opportunity in the absence of some account of what it could mean for these things to be practically realized. Discussions about political philosophy and health policy need to be combined and to inform one another. Finally, I would suggest, these discussions can no more be left to experts than can discussions about healthcare be left to health professionals. If we are concerned about equal respect, both respect for ourselves and for one another, we each have a job to do (even if only on our doorstep). The goods of health are not products which some individuals provide to others. They are goods that we are all responsible for shaping and securing.

Bibliography

Appadurai, A. (1996). *Modernity at Large: Cultural Dimensions of Globalisation*. Minneapolis: University of Minnesota Press.

Apple, M. W. (1993). *Official Knowledge: Democratic Education in a Conservative Age*. New York: Routledge.

Arnstein, S. (1971). 'Eight rungs on the ladder of citizen participation', in E. S. Cahn and B. A. Passett (eds.), *Citizen Participation*. London: Praeger.

Barber, N. D. (1991). Is 'safe, effective and economic' enough? *Pharmaceutical Journal*, 246: 671–2.

Barnett, R. (1994). University knowledge in an age of supercomplexity. *Higher Education*, 40: 409–22.

Beaglehole, R., and Bonita, R. (1997). *Public Health at the Crossroads*. Cambridge: Cambridge University Press.

Beattie, A. (1991). 'Knowledge and control in health promotion: a test case for social policy and social theory', in Gabe, J., Calnan, M., and Bury, M. (eds.), *The Sociology of the Health Service*. London: Routledge.

Beauchamp, T. L., and Childress, J. F. (2001). *Principles of Biomedical Ethics*. Oxford: Oxford University Press.

Benner, P., and Wrubel, J. (1989). *The Primacy of Caring: Stress and Coping in Health and Illness*. Menlo Park, Calif.: Addison-Wesley.

Berg, M. (2001). Guidelines for Appropriate Care: The Importance of Empirical Normative Analysis. *Health Care Analysis*, 9/1: 77–99.

Boorse, C. (1977). Health as a Theoretical Concept. *Philosophy of Science*, 44: 542–573.

Bourdieu, P. (1986). 'The Forms of Capital', in J. G. Richardson (ed.). *Handbook of Theory and Research for the Sociology of Education*. New York: Greenwood Press.

Bowden, P. (1997). *Caring: Gender-Sensitive Ethics*. London: Routledge.

Brock, D. W. (1987). Truth or Consequences: The Role of Philosophy in Policy Making. *Ethics*, 97: 786–91.

Brülde, B. (2001). The Goals of Medicine. Towards a Unified Theory. *Health Care Analysis*, 9/1: 1–13.

Bunton, R., Nettleton, S., and Burrows, R. (1995). *The Sociology of Health Promotion: Critical Analyses of Consumption, Lifestyle and Risk*. London: Routledge.

Burr, V. (1995). *An Introduction to Social Constructionism*. London: Routledge.

Callahan, D. (1990). *What Kind of Life: The Limits of Medical Progress*. Washington DC: Georgetown University Press.

Callahan, J. (1998). *Ethical Issues in Professional Life*. Oxford: Oxford University Press.

Campbell, A. V. (1984). *Moderated Love: A Theology of Professional Care*. London: SPCK.

—— (1990). 'Education or Indoctrination? The issue of autonomy in health education', in S. Doxiadis (ed.), *Ethics in Health Education*. Chichester: John Wiley &
Sons.

—— (2000). 'My country tis of thee'—the Myopia of American Bioethics. *Medicine,
Health Care and Philosophy, 3/2: 195–8.*

Caplan, R., and Holland, R. (1990). Rethinking health education theory. *Health
Education Journal*, 49/1: 10–12.

Charles, C., Gafni, A., and Whelan, T. (1997). Shared decision-making in the medical
encounter: what does it mean? *Social Science and Medicine*, 44: 681–92.

Clarke, J., and Newman, J. (1997). *The Managerial State*. London: Sage.

Cribb, A. (2002). 'Ethics: from health care to public policy', in L. Jones & M. Siddel
(eds.), *The Challenge of Promoting Health: Exploration and Action*. London: Macmillan.

—— and Gewirtz, S. (2003). 'Towards a Sociology of Just Practices', in Vincent C.
(ed.), *Social Justice, Education and Identity*. London: Routledge Falmer.

Daniels, N. (1985). *Just Health Care*. Cambridge: Cambridge University Press.

—— and Sabin, J. (1998). Ethics of accountability in managed care reform. *Health
Affairs*, 17: 50–64.

Del Vecchio Good, M., Munakata, T., Kobawashi, Y., Mattingly, C., and Good, B.
(1994). Oncology and narrative time. *Social Science and Medicine*, 38/6: 855–62.

Department of Health (2000). *Department of Health Guidance on Tackling Teenage
Pregnancy*. London: Dept. of Health Teenage Pregnancy Unit, Dept. of Health.

Dickenson, D. (1999). Can Medical Criteria Settle Priority-Setting Debates? The
Need for Ethical Analysis. *Health Care Analysis*, 7/1: 1–7.

—— and Vineis, P. (2002). Evidence-Based Medicine and Quality of Care. *Health
Care Analysis*, 10/3: 243–59.

Dines, A. (1997). 'A Case Study of Ethical Issues in Health Promotion–Mammog-
raphy Screening: The Nurse's Position', in Siddell, M., Jones, L., Katz, J., and
Peberdy, A. (eds.), *Debates and Dilemmas in Promoting Health*. Basingstoke: Macmillan.

Donovan, G. K. (2000). 'The Physician-Patient Relationship' in Thomasma, D. C.,
and Kissell, J. L. (eds.), *The Health Care Professional as Friend and Healer*.
Washington DC: Georgetown University Press.

Downie, R. S., Tannahill, C., and Tannahill, A. (1996). *Health Promotion: Models
and Values*. Oxford: Oxford University Press.

Doyal, L. (1998). Public participation and the moral quality of healthcare rationing.
Quality in Health Care, 7: 98–102.

—— and Gough, I. (1986) *A Theory of Human Needs*. London: Macmillan.

Dworkin, R. (1977). *Taking Rights Seriously*. London: Duckworth.

—— (1981). Voluntary health risks and public policy. *Hastings Center Report*, 11/5:
26–31.

—— (2000). *Sovereign Virtue: The Theory and Practice of Equality.* Cambridge,
Mass.: Harvard University Press.

Easton, D. (1953). *The Political System: An inquiry into the state of political science*.
New York: Knopf.

Eraut, M. (1994). *Developing Professional Knowledge and Competence*. London: Falmer Press.

Erin, C. A., and Harris, J. (1993). AIDS: Ethics, Justice and Social Policy. *Journal of Applied Philosophy*, 10/2: 165–73.

Ewles, L., and Simnett, I. (1995). *Promoting Health: A Practical Guide to Health Education*. Harrow: Scutari Press.

Fay, B. (1975). *Social theory and political practice*. London: Allen & Unwin.

Freidson, E. (2001). *Professionalism: the Third Logic*. Cambridge: Polity Press.

Flyvbjerg, B. (2001). *Making Social Science Matter: Why Social Inquiry Fails and How it Can Succeed Again*. Cambridge: Cambridge University Press.

Forbes, A., and Wainwright, S. P. (2001). On the methodological, theoretical, philosophical and political context of health inequalities research: A critique. *Social Science & Medicine*, 53: 801–16.

Foucault, M. (1978). *The History of Sexuality, Vol. 1: An Introduction*. New York: Random House.

Fraser, N. (1977). *Justice Interruptus: Critical Reflections on the 'Postsocialist' Condition*. London: Routledge.

Frith, L. (2002). 'Clinical Governance. An Ethical Perspective–Quality and Judgement', in Tingle, J., and Cribb, A. (eds.), *Nursing Law and Ethics*. Oxford: Blackwell.

Giddens, A. (1984). *The Constitution of Society–Outline of the Theory of Structuration*. Cambridge: Polity Press.

—— (1991). *Modernity and Self-Identity, Self and Society in the Late Modern Age*. Cambridge: Polity Press.

Goodin, R. (1989). *No Smoking—The Ethical Issues*. Chicago: University of Chicago Press.

Graham, H. (ed.). (2000). *Understanding Health Inequalities*. Buckingham: Open University Press.

Griffin, J. (1986). *Well-being. Its Meaning, Measurement and Moral Importance*. Oxford: Clarendon Press.

—— (1996). *Value Judgement. Improving Our Ethical Beliefs*. Oxford: Clarendon Press.

Gutmann, A., and Thompson, D. (1996). *Democracy and Disagreement*. Cambridge, Mass.: Harvard University Press.

Hall, S. (1998). The Great Moving Nowhere Show. *Marxism Today*, Nov.–Dec.: 9–14.

Hardwig, J. (2000). *Is There a Duty to Die? And Other Essays in Bioethics*. London and New York: Routledge.

Hirst, P., and Thompson, G. (1999). *Globalization in Question: The International Economy and the Possibilities of Governance*. Cambridge: Polity Press.

Holm, S. (1998). Goodbye to the simple solutions: the second phase of priority setting in health care. *British Medical Journal*, 7164: 1000–2.

Hoyle, E. (1980). 'Professionalisation and deprofessionalisation in education', in E. Hoyle and J. Megarry (eds)., World Yearbook of Education 1980. London: Kogan Page.

Humber, J. M., and Almeder R. F. (eds.) (2000). *Is There a Duty to Die? Biomedical Ethics Reviews*. Totowa, NJ: Humana Press.

Khushf, G. (2000). 'Organizational Ethics and the Medical Professional: Reappraising Roles and Responsibilities', in Thomasma, D. C., and Kissell, J. L. (eds.), *The Health Care Professional as Friend and Healer*. Washington, DC: Georgetown University Press.

—— (2001). What is at Issue in the Debate about Concepts of Health and Disease? Framing the Problem of Demarcation for a Post-positivist Era of Medicine, in L. Nordenfelt (ed.), *Health, Science and Ordinary Language*. Amsterdam/Atlanta, GA: Rodopi.

—— and McKeown, R. (2000). A Schema of Health Concepts: Clarifying Values in Public Health Strategic Planning. Unpublished Report.

Koehn, D. (1994). *The Ground of Professional Ethics*. London: Routledge.

Le Grand, J., and Bartlett, W. (1993) *Quasi-Markets and Social Policy*. London: Macmillan.

Lewis, G., Gewirtz, S., and Clarke J. (eds.) (2000). *Rethinking Social Policy*, London: Sage.

Lomas, J. (1997). Reluctant rationers: public input to health care priorities. *Journal of Health Service Research Policy*, 2/2: 1–8.

MacIntyre, A. (1985). *After Virtue–A Study in Moral Theory*. London: Duckworth.

McKinlay, J. B. (2001). 'A Case for Refocusing Upstream: The Political Economy of Illness', in Conrad, P. (ed.), *The Sociology of Health and Illness: Critical Perspectives*. 6th edn., New York: Worth Publishers.

Maclean, A. (1993). *The Elimination of Morality: Reflections on Utilitarianism and Bioethics*. London: Routledge.

Martin, D., and Singer, P. (2003). A Strategy to Improve Priority Setting in Health Care Institutions. *Health Care Analysis*, 11/1: 59–68.

Massey, D. (1999). 'Imagining globalization: power-geometries of time-space', in A. Brah, M. Hickman and M. Mac an Ghaill (eds)., *Future Worlds: Migration, Environment and Globalization*. London: Macmillan.

Mill, J. S. (1948). *On Liberty and Considerations on Representative Government*. Oxford : Blackwell.

Millar, R., and Osborne, J. F. (eds.) (1998). *Beyond 2000: Science Education for the Future*. London: King's College London.

Molewijk, A. C., Stiggelbout, A. M., Otten, W., Dupuis, H. M., and Kievit, J. (2003). Implicit Normativity in Evidence-Based Medicine: A Plea for Integrated Empirical Ethics Research. *Health Care Analysis*, 11/1: 69–92.

Nettleton, S. (1995). *The Sociology of Health and Illness*. Cambridge: Polity Press.

Nord, E. (1999). Towards Cost-Value Analysis in Health Care? *Health Care Analysis*, 7/2: 167–75.

Nordenfelt, L. (1987). *On the Nature of Health*. Dordrecht: D. Reidel.

—— (1998). On Medicine and Other Means of Health Enhancement—Towards a Conceptual Framework. *Medicine, Health Care and Philosophy*, 1: 5–12.

Norman, I., and Cowley, S. (1998). *The Changing Nature of Nursing in a Managerial Age*. Oxford: Blackwell.

Oakeshott, M. (1962). The Tower of Babel. In *Rationalism in Politics*. London: Methuen.

Parsons, T. (1981). 'Definitions of health and illness in the light of American values and social structure', in A. L. Caplan, H. T. Englehardt, Jr & J.J. McCartney (eds.), *Concepts of Health and Disease: Interdisciplinary Perspectives*. Reading, Mass.: Addison-Wesley.

Pateman, C. (1970). Participation and Democratic Theory. Cambridge: Cambridge University Press.

Peters, R. S. (1966). *Ethics and Education*. London: Allen & Unwin.

—— (1981). Reason and Habit: The Paradox of Moral Education. *In Moral Development and Moral Education*. London: Allen & Unwin.

Plant, R., and Barry, N. (1990) *Citizenship and Rights in Thatcher's Britain: Two Views*. London: Institute of Economic Affairs.

—— Lesser, H., and Taylor-Gooby, P. (1980). *Political Philosophy and Social Welfare: Essays on the Normative Basis of Welfare Provision*. London: Routledge & Kegan Paul.

Radley, A. (1993). *Worlds of Illness: Biographical and Cultural Perspectives on Health and Disease*. London: Routledge.

Rawls, J. (1972). *A Theory of Justice*. Oxford: Clarendon Press.

Raz, J. (1994). *Ethics in the Public Domain*. Oxford: Clarendon Press.

Rose, N. (1996). 'Governing "advanced" liberal democracies', in A. Barry, T. Osborne, and N. Rose (eds.). *Foucault and Political Reason: Liberalism, Neo-Liberalism and Rationalities of Government*. London: UCL Press.

Royal Pharmaceutical Society (1997). *From Compliance to Concordance. Achieving Shared Goals in Medicine Taking*. London: Royal Pharmaceutical Society and Merck, Sharpe & Dohme.

Sackett, D. L., Rosenberg, W. M., Muir Gray, J. A., Haynes, R. B., and Richardson, W. S. (1996). Evidence based medicine: what it is and what it isn't. *British Medical Journal*, 312: 71–2.

Searle, J. (1995). *The Construction of Social Reality*. New York: Free Press.

Seedhouse, D. (2001). *Health. The Foundations for Achievement*. Chichester: John Wiley & Sons.

Sivanandan, A. (1989). New Circuits of Imperialism. *Race & Class*, 30/4: 1–19.

Sorell, T. (2001). Citizen-Patient/Citizen-Doctor. *Health Care Analysis*, 9/1: 25–39.

Sumner, L. W. (1996). *Welfare, Happiness and Ethics*. Oxford: Clarendon Press.

Taylor, C. (1992). *The Ethics of Authenticity*. Cambridge, Mass.: Harvard University Press.

Tones, K. (2002). Reveille for Radicals! The Paramount Purpose of Health Education? *Health Education Research*, 17/1: 1–6.

—— and Tilford, S. (2001). *Health Education: Effectiveness, Efficiency and Equity*. London: Chapman Hall.

Veatch, R. M. (1987). *The Patient as Partner*. Bloomington: Indiana University Press.

—— (2000). *Transplantation Ethics*. Washington, DC: Georgetown University Press.

Wenger, E. (1998). *Communities of Practice: Learning, Meaning and Identity*. Cambridge: Cambridge University Press.

Whitehead, M., Diderichsen, F., and Burström, B. (2000). 'Researching the impact of public policy on inequalities in health', in H. Graham (ed.), *Understanding Health Inequalities*. Buckingham: Open University Press.

WHO (World Health Organization) (1946). *Constitution*. New York: World Health Organization.

—— (1977). *Global Strategy for Health for All by the Year 2000*. Geneva: World Health Organization.

—— (1986). *Ottowa Charter for Health Promotion*. Geneva: World Health Organization.

Wikler, D. (1978). Persuasion and coercion for health: ethical issues in government efforts to change lifestyles. *Millbank Memorial Fund Quarterly/ Health and Society*, 56/3: 303–38.

—— (1987). Who should be blamed for being sick? *Health Education Quarterly*, 14/1: 11–25.

Wilkinson, R. (1996). *Unhealthy Societies: The Afflictions of Inequality*. London: Routledge.

Wilkinson, S. (1999). Smokers' Rights to Health Care: Why the 'Restoration Argument' is a Moralising Wolf in a Liberal Sheep's Clothing. *Journal of Applied Philosophy*, 16/3: 255–69.

Williams, G. (1989). 'The genesis of chronic illness: narrative reconstruction', in Brown, P. (ed.), *Perspectives in Medical Sociology*. Belmont, Calif.: Wadsworth.

Winch, P. (1958). *The Idea of a Social Science and its Relation to Philosophy*. London: Routledge & Kegan Paul.

Wirtz, V., Cribb, A., and Barber, N. (2003). Understanding the Role of 'The Hidden Curriculum' in Resource Allocation—The Case of the UK NHS. *Health Care Analysis*, 11/4: 295–300.

Wiseman, V. (1999). Culture, Self-Rated Health and Resource Allocation Decision-Making. *Health Care Analysis*, 7/3: 207–23.

Wong, K. L. (2000). *Medicine and the Marketplace. The Moral Dimensions of Managed Care*. Notre Dame, Ind.: University of Notre Dame Press.

Yeatman, A. (1987). The Concept of Public Management and the Australian State in the 1980s. *Australian Journal of Public Administration*, XLVI/4: 334–53.

Young, I. M. (1990). *Justice and the Politics of Difference*. Princeton, NJ: Princeton University Press.

Index